WHO/BTS/99
Distr. General
Orig.: English

# The
# Clinical
# Use
# of
# Blood

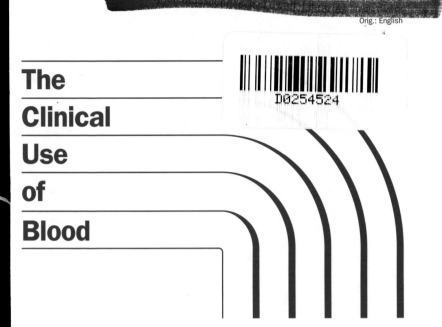

## Handbook

**World Health Organization**
**Blood Transfusion Safety**
GENEVA

WHO Library Cataloguing-in-Publication Data

The clinical use of blood: handbook.

1. Blood transfusion - handbooks  2. Plasma  3. Anemia - therapy
4. Anemia - in infancy and childhood  5. Pregnancy complications - therapy  6. Intraoperative complications - therapy
7. Wounds and injuries - therapy  8. Burns - therapy

ISBN 92 4 154539 9          (NLM classification: WH 460)

Printed in Malta

**The Clinical Use of Blood: handbook**
Sw.fr. 15.–
In developing countries: Sw.fr. 10.50

ISBN 92 4 154539 9

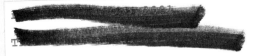

# Contents

# Preface

Blood transfusion is an essential part of modern health care. Used correctly, it can save life and improve health. However, the transmission of infectious agents by blood and blood products has focused particular attention on the potential risks of transfusion.

The World Health Organization (WHO) has developed the following integrated strategies to promote global blood safety and minimize the risks associated with transfusion.

1   The establishment of nationally-coordinated blood transfusion services with quality systems in all areas.

2   The collection of blood only from voluntary non-remunerated blood donors from low-risk populations.

3   The screening of all donated blood for transfusion-transmissible infections, including the human immunodeficiency virus (HIV), hepatitis viruses, syphilis and other infectious agents, and good laboratory practice in all aspects of blood grouping, compatibility testing, component preparation and the storage and transportation of blood and blood products.

4   A reduction in unnecessary transfusions through the appropriate clinical use of blood and blood products, and the use of simple alternatives to transfusion, wherever possible.

In support of these strategies, WHO has produced a series of recommendations, guidelines and learning materials, including Recommendations on *Developing a National Policy and Guidelines on the Clinical Use of Blood*. This document was designed to assist Member States in developing and implementing national policies and guidelines and ensuring active collaboration between the blood transfusion service and clinicians throughout the management of patients who may require transfusion.

The Recommendations emphasize the importance of education and training in the clinical use of blood for all clinical and blood bank staff involved in the transfusion process.

The WHO team responsible for Blood Transfusion Safety (WHO/BTS) has therefore developed a module of interactive learning material, *The Clinical Use of Blood*, that can be used in undergraduate and postgraduate programmes, in-service training and continuing medical education programmes or for independent study by individual clinicians and blood transfusion specialists. The module is available from WHO Distribution & Sales and WHO Regional Offices.

This pocket handbook summarizes the information contained in the module and has been produced for quick reference by clinicians who need to make urgent decisions on transfusion.

The module and handbook have been written by an international team of clinical and blood transfusion medicine specialists and have been reviewed by a wide range of specialists throughout the world. They have also been reviewed by the WHO Departments of Reproductive Health and Research, Child and Adolescent Health and Development, Management of Non-Communicable Diseases (Human Genetics) and Roll Back Malaria.

Nevertheless, clinical transfusion practice should always be based on national guidelines, where available. You are therefore encouraged to adapt the information and guidance contained in this handbook to conform with national guidelines and established procedures in your own country.

**Dr Jean C. Emmanuel**
**Director, Blood Safety & Clinical Technology**
**World Health Organization**

# Introduction

*The Clinical Use of Blood* forms part of a series of learning materials developed by WHO/BTS in support of its global strategy for blood safety. It focuses on the clinical aspects of blood transfusion and aims to show how unnecessary transfusions can be reduced at all levels of the health care system in any country, without compromising standards of quality and safety.

It contains two components:

- A module of learning material designed for use in education and training programmes or for independent study by individual clinicians and blood transfusion specialists
- A pocket handbook for use in clinical practice.

## The module

The module is designed for prescribers of blood at all levels of the health system, particularly clinicians and senior paramedical staff at first referral level (district hospitals) in developing countries.

It provides a comprehensive guide to the use of blood and blood products and, in particular, ways of minimizing unnecessary transfusion.

## The handbook

The pocket handbook summarizes key information from the module to provide a quick reference when an urgent decision on transfusion is required.

It is important to follow national guidelines on clinical blood use if they differ in any way from the guidance contained in the module and handbook. You may therefore find it useful to add your own notes on national guidelines or your own experience in prescribing transfusion.

## The evidence base for clinical practice

*The Clinical Use of Blood* has been prepared by an international team of clinical and blood transfusion specialists and has been extensively reviewed by relevant WHO departments and by Critical Readers from a range of clinical disciplines from all six of the WHO regions. The content reflects the knowledge and experience of the contributors and reviewers. However, since the evidence for effective clinical practice is constantly evolving, you are encouraged to consult up-to-date sources of information such as the Cochrane Library, the National Library of Medicine database and the WHO Reproductive Health Library.

**The Cochrane Library.** Systematic reviews of the effects of health care interventions, available on diskette, CD-ROM and via the Internet. There are Cochrane Centres in Africa, Asia, Australasia, Europe, North America and South America. For information, contact: UK Cochrane Centre, NHS Research and Development Programme, Summertown Pavilion, Middle Way, Oxford OX2 7LG, UK. Tel: +44 1865 516300. Fax: +44 1865 516311. www.cochrane.org

**National Library of Medicine**. An online biomedical library, including *Medline* which contains references and abstracts from 4300 biomedical journals and *Clinical Trials* which provides information on clinical research studies. National Library of Medicine, 8600 Rockville Pike, Bethesda, MD 20894, USA. www.nlm.nih.gov

**WHO Reproductive Health Library**. An electronic review journal focusing on evidence-based solutions to reproductive health problems in developing countries. Available on CD-ROM from Reproductive Health and Research, World Health Organization, 1211 Geneva 27, Switzerland. www.who.int

# The appropriate use of blood and blood products

## Key points

1 The appropriate use of blood and blood products means the transfusion of safe blood products only to treat a condition leading to significant morbidity or mortality that cannot be prevented or managed effectively by other means.

2 Transfusion carries the risk of adverse reactions and transfusion-transmissible infections. Plasma can transmit most of the infections present in whole blood and there are very few indications for its transfusion.

3 Blood donated by family/replacement donors carries a higher risk of transfusion-transmissible infections than blood donated by voluntary non-remunerated donors. Paid blood donors generally have the highest incidence and prevalence of transfusion-transmissible infections.

4 Blood should not be transfused unless it has been obtained from appropriately selected donors, has been screened for transfusion-transmissible infections and tested for compatibility between the donor's red cells and the antibodies in the patient's plasma, in accordance with national requirements.

5 The need for transfusion can often be avoided by:
- The prevention or early diagnosis and treatment of anaemia and conditions that cause anaemia
- The correction of anaemia and the replacement of depleted iron stores before planned surgery
- The use of simple alternatives to transfusion, such as intravenous replacement fluids
- Good anaesthetic and surgical management.

# Appropriate and inappropriate transfusion

Blood transfusion can be a life-saving intervention. However, like all treatments, it may result in acute or delayed complications and carries the risk of transfusion-transmissible infections, including HIV, hepatitis viruses, syphilis, malaria and Chagas disease.

The safety and effectiveness of transfusion depend on two key factors:

- A supply of blood and blood products that are safe, accessible at reasonable cost and adequate to meet national needs
- The appropriate clinical use of blood and blood products.

Transfusion is often unnecessary for the following reasons.

1 The need for transfusion can often be avoided or minimized by the prevention or early diagnosis and treatment of anaemia and conditions that cause anaemia.

2 Blood is often unnecessarily given to raise a patient's haemoglobin level before surgery or to allow earlier discharge from hospital. These are rarely valid reasons for transfusion.

3 Transfusions of whole blood, red cells or plasma are often given when other treatments, such as the infusion of normal saline or other intravenous replacement fluids would be safer, less expensive and equally effective for the treatment of acute blood loss.

4 Patients' transfusion requirements can often be minimized by good anaesthetic and surgical management.

5 If blood is given when it is not needed, the patient receives no benefit and is exposed to unnecessary risk.

6 Blood is an expensive, scarce resource. Unnecessary transfusions may cause a shortage of blood products for patients in real need.

## The risks of transfusion

In some clinical situations, transfusion may be the only way to save life or rapidly improve a serious condition. However, before prescribing blood or blood products for a patient, it is always essential to weigh up the risks of transfusion against the risks of not transfusing.

### Red cell transfusion

1 The transfusion of red cell products carries a risk of serious haemolytic transfusion reactions.

2 Blood products can transmit infectious agents, including HIV, hepatitis B, hepatitis C, syphilis, malaria and Chagas disease to the recipient.

3 Any blood product can become contaminated with bacteria and very dangerous if it is manufactured or stored incorrectly.

### Plasma transfusion

1 Plasma can transmit most of the infections present in whole blood.

2 Plasma can also cause transfusion reactions.

3 There are few clear clinical indications for plasma transfusion. The risks very often outweigh any possible benefit to the patient.

## Blood safety

The quality and safety of all blood and blood products must be assured throughout the process from the selection of blood donors through to their administration to the patient. This requires:

1 The establishment of a well-organized blood transfusion service with quality systems in all areas.

2 The collection of blood only from voluntary non-remunerated donors from low-risk populations and rigorous procedures for donor selection.

3 The screening of all donated blood for transfusion-transmissible infections: HIV, hepatitis viruses, syphilis and, where appropriate, other infectious agents, such as Chagas disease and malaria.

4 Good laboratory practice in all aspects of blood grouping, compatibility testing, component preparation and the storage and transportation of blood and blood products.

5 A reduction in unnecessary transfusions through the appropriate clinical use of blood and blood products, and the use of simple alternatives to transfusion, wherever possible.

Other than in the most exceptional life-threatening situations, blood should not be issued for transfusion unless it has been obtained from appropriately selected donors and has been screened for transfusion-transmissible infections, in accordance with national requirements.

Whatever the local system for the collection, screening and processing of blood, clinicians must be familiar with it and understand any limitations that it may impose on the safety or availability of blood.

## Principles of clinical transfusion practice

Transfusion is only one part of the patient's management. The need for transfusion can often be minimized by the following means.

1 The prevention or early diagnosis and treatment of anaemia and the conditions that cause anaemia. The patient's haemoglobin level can often be raised by iron and vitamin supplementation without the need for transfusion. Red cell transfusion is needed only if the effects of chronic anaemia are severe enough to require rapid raising of the haemoglobin level.

2 The correction of anaemia and replacement of depleted iron stores before planned surgery.

3 The use of intravenous fluid replacement with crystalloids or colloids in cases of acute blood loss.

4 Good anaesthetic and surgical management, including:
   - Using the best anaesthetic and surgical techniques to minimize blood loss during surgery
   - Stopping anticoagulants and anti-platelet drugs before planned surgery, where it is safe to do so
   - Minimizing the blood taken for laboratory use, particularly in children
   - Salvaging and reinfusing surgical blood losses
   - Using alternative approaches such as desmopressin, aprotinin or erythropoetin.

## PRINCIPLES OF CLINICAL TRANSFUSION PRACTICE

1  Transfusion is only one part of the patient's management.

2  Prescribing should be based on national guidelines on the clinical use of blood, taking individual patient needs into account.

3  Blood loss should be minimized to reduce the patient's need for transfusion.

4  The patient with acute blood loss should receive effective resuscitation (intravenous replacement fluids, oxygen, etc.) while the need for transfusion is being assessed.

5  The patient's haemoglobin value, although important, should not be the sole deciding factor in starting transfusion. This decision should be supported by the need to relieve clinical signs and symptoms and prevent significant morbidity or mortality.

6  The clinician should be aware of the risks of transfusion-transmissible infections in the blood products that are available for the individual patient.

7  Transfusion should be prescribed only when the benefits to the patient are likely to outweigh the risks.

8  The clinician should record the reason for transfusion clearly.

9  A trained person should monitor the transfused patient and respond immediately if any adverse effects occur.

# Notes

# Replacement fluids

1  Replacement fluids are used to replace abnormal losses of blood, plasma or other extracellular fluids by increasing the volume of the vascular compartment, principally in:
   - Treatment of patients with established hypovolaemia: e.g. haemorrhagic shock
   - Maintenance of normovolaemia in patients with ongoing fluid losses: e.g. surgical blood loss.

2  Intravenous replacement fluids are the first-line treatment for hypovolaemia. Initial treatment with these fluids may be life-saving and provide some time to control bleeding and obtain blood for transfusion, if it becomes necessary.

3  Crystalloid solutions with a similar concentration of sodium to plasma (normal saline or balanced salt solutions) are effective as replacement fluids. Dextrose (glucose) solutions do not contain sodium and are poor replacement fluids.

4  Crystalloid replacement fluids should be infused in a volume at least three times the volume lost in order to correct hypovolaemia.

5  All colloid solutions (albumin, dextrans, gelatins and hydroxyethyl starch solutions) are replacement fluids. However, they have not been shown to be superior to crystalloids in resuscitation.

6  Colloid solutions should be infused in a volume equal to the blood volume deficit.

7  Plasma should never be used as a replacement fluid.

8  Plain water should never be infused intravenously. It will cause haemolysis and will probably be fatal.

9  In addition to the intravenous route, the intraosseous, oral, rectal or subcutaneous routes can be used for the administration of fluids.

## Intravenous replacement therapy

The administration of intravenous replacement fluids restores the circulating blood volume and so maintains tissue perfusion and oxygenation.

In severe haemorrhage, initial treatment (resuscitation) with intravenous replacement fluids may be life-saving and provide time to control the bleeding and order blood for transfusion, if necessary.

## Intravenous replacement fluids

### Crystalloid solutions

- Contain a similar concentration of sodium to plasma
- Are excluded from the intracellular compartment because the cell membrane is generally impermeable to sodium
- Cross the capillary membrane from the vascular compartment to the interstitial compartment
- Are distributed through the whole extracellular compartment
- Normally, only a quarter of the volume of crystalloid infused remains in the vascular compartment.

### COMPOSITION OF CRYSTALLOID REPLACEMENT SOLUTIONS

| Fluid | $Na^+$ mmol/L | $K^+$ mmol/L | $Ca^{2+}$ mmol/L | $Cl^-$ mmol/L | Base$^-$ mEq/L | Colloid osmotic pressure mmHg |
|---|---|---|---|---|---|---|
| Normal saline (sodium chloride 0.9%) | 154 | 0 | 0 | 154 | 0 | 0 |
| Balanced salt solutions (Ringer's lactate or Hartmann's solution) | 130–140 | 4–5 | 2–3 | 109–110 | 28–30 | 0 |

To restore circulating blood volume (intravascular volume), crystalloid solutions should be infused in a volume at least three times the volume lost.

> Dextrose (glucose) solutions do not contain sodium and are poor replacement fluids. Do not use to treat hypovolaemia unless there is no alternative.

## Colloid solutions

- Initially tend to remain within the vascular compartment
- Mimic plasma proteins, thereby maintaining or raising the colloid osmotic pressure of blood
- Provide longer duration of plasma volume expansion than crystalloid solutions
- Require smaller infusion volumes.

### COMPOSITION OF COLLOID REPLACEMENT SOLUTIONS

| Fluid | $Na^+$ mmol/L | $K^+$ mmol/L | $Ca^{2+}$ mmol/L | $Cl^-$ mmol/L | $Base^-$ mEq/L | Colloid osmotic pressure mmHg |
|---|---|---|---|---|---|---|
| Gelatin (urea linked): e.g. Haemaccel | 145 | 5.1 | 6.25 | 145 | Trace amounts | 27 |
| Gelatin (succinylated): e.g. Gelofusine | 154 | <0.4 | <0.4 | 125 | Trace amounts | 34 |
| Dextran 70 (6%) | 154 | 0 | 0 | 154 | 0 | 58 |
| Dextran 60 (3%) | 130 | 4 | 2 | 110 | 30 | 22 |
| Hydroxyethyl starch 450/0.7 (6%) | 154 | 0 | 0 | 154 | 0 | 28 |
| Albumin 5% | 130–160 | <1 | V | V | V | 27 |
| Ionic composition of normal plasma | 135–145 | 3.5–5.5 | 2.2–2.6 | 97–110 | 38–44 | 27 |

V = varies between different brands

> Colloids require smaller infusion volumes than crystalloids. They are usually given in a volume equal to the blood volume deficit.

However, when the capillary permeability is increased, they may leak from the circulation and produce only a short-lived volume expansion.

Supplementary infusions will be needed to maintain blood volume in conditions such as:

- Trauma
- Acute and chronic sepsis
- Burns
- Snake bite (haemotoxic and cytotoxic).

|  | Advantages | Disadvantages |
|---|---|---|
| **Crystalloids** | ■ Few side-effects<br>■ Low cost<br>■ Wide availability | ■ Short duration of action<br>■ May cause oedema<br>■ Weighty and bulky |
| **Colloids** | ■ Longer duration of action<br>■ Less fluid required to correct hypovolaemia<br>■ Less weighty and bulky | ■ No evidence that they are more clinically effective<br>■ Higher cost<br>■ May cause volume overload<br>■ May interfere with clotting<br>■ Risk of anaphylactic reactions |

**There is no evidence that colloid solutions are superior to normal saline (sodium chloride 0.9%) or balanced salt solutions (BSS) for resuscitation.**

## Maintenance fluids

- Used to replace normal physiological losses through skin, lung, faeces and urine
- The volume of maintenance fluids required by a patient will vary, particularly with pyrexia, high ambient temperature or humidity, when losses will increase
- Composed mainly of water in a dextrose solution; may contain some electrolytes
- All maintenance fluids are crystalloid solutions.

### Examples of maintenance fluids

- 5% dextrose
- 4% dextrose in sodium chloride 0.18%.

## Safety

Before giving any intravenous infusion:

1 Check that the seal of the infusion bottle or bag is not broken.

2 Check the expiry date.

3 Check that the solution is clear and free from visible particles.

## Other routes of fluid administration

There are other routes of fluid administration in addition to the intravenous route. However, with the exception of the intraosseous route, they are generally unsuitable in the severely hypovolaemic patient.

### Intraosseous

- Can provide the quickest access to the circulation in a shocked child in whom venous cannulation is impossible
- Fluids, blood and certain drugs can be administered by this route
- Suitable in the severely hypovolaemic patient.

### Oral and nasogastric

- Can often be used in patients who are mildly hypovolaemic and in whom the oral route is not contraindicated
- Should not be used in patients if:
  — Severely hypovolaemic
  — Unconscious
  — Gastrointestinal lesions or reduced gut motility
  — General anaesthesia and surgery is planned imminently.

---

**WHO/UNICEF formula for oral rehydration fluid**

**Dissolve in one litre of potable water**

| | |
|---|---|
| Sodium chloride (table salt) | 3.5 g |
| Sodium bicarbonate (baking soda) | 2.5 g |
| Potassium chloride or substitute (banana or degassed cola drink) | 1.5 g |
| Glucose (sugar) | 20.0 g |

**Resulting concentrations**

$Na^+$ 90 mmol/L   $K^+$ 20 mmol/L   $Cl^-$ 80 mmol/L   Glucose 110 mmol/L

---

## Rectal

- Unsuitable in the severely hypovolaemic patient
- Ready absorption of fluids
- Absorption ceases with fluids being ejected when hydration is complete
- Administered through plastic or rubber enema tube inserted into the rectum and connected to a bag or bottle of fluid
- Fluid rate can be controlled by using a drip infusion set, if necessary
- Fluids used do not have to be sterile: a safe and effective solution for rectal rehydration is 1 litre of clean drinking water to which is added a teaspoon of table salt.

## Subcutaneous

- Can occasionally be used when other routes of administration of fluids are unavailable
- Unsuitable in the severely hypovolaemic patient
- A cannula or needle is inserted into the subcutaneous tissue (the abdominal wall is a preferred site) and sterile fluids are administered in a conventional manner
- Dextrose-containing solutions can cause sloughing of tissues and should not be given subcutaneously.

# Crystalloid solutions

## NORMAL SALINE (Sodium chloride 0.9%)

| | |
|---|---|
| Infection risk | Nil |
| Indications | Replacement of blood volume and other extracellular fluid losses |
| Precautions | ■ Caution in situations where local oedema may aggravate pathology: e.g. head injury<br>■ May precipitate volume overload and heart failure |
| Contraindications | Do not use in patients with established renal failure |
| Side-effects | Tissue oedema can develop when large volumes are used |
| Dosage | At least 3 times the blood volume lost |

## BALANCED SALT SOLUTIONS

| | |
|---|---|
| Examples | ■ Ringer's lactate<br>■ Hartmann's solution |
| Infection risk | Nil |
| Indications | Replacement of blood volume and other extracellular fluid losses |
| Precautions | ■ Caution in situations where local oedema may aggravate pathology: e.g. head injury<br>■ May precipitate volume overload and heart failure |
| Contraindications | Do not use in patients with established renal failure |
| Side-effects | Tissue oedema can develop when large volumes are used |
| Dosage | At least 3 times the blood volume lost |

## DEXTROSE and ELECTROLYTE SOLUTIONS

| | |
|---|---|
| Examples | ■ 4.3% dextrose in sodium chloride 0.18% |
| | ■ 2.5% dextrose in sodium chloride 0.45% |
| | ■ 2.5% dextrose in half-strength Darrow's solution |
| Indications | Generally used for maintenance fluids, but those containing higher concentrations of sodium can, if necessary, be used as replacement fluids |

**Note**

2.5% dextrose in half-strength Darrow's solution is commonly used to correct dehydration and electrolyte disturbances in children with gastroenteritis

Several products are manufactured for this use. Not all are suitable. Ensure that the preparation you use contains:

■ Dextrose    2.5%
■ Sodium      60 mmol/L
■ Potassium   17 mmol/L
■ Chloride    52 mmol/L
■ Lactate     25 mmol/L

# Plasma-derived (natural) colloid solutions

Plasma-derived colloids are all prepared from donated blood or plasma. They include:

- Plasma
- Fresh frozen plasma
- Liquid plasma
- Freeze-dried plasma
- Albumin

**These products should not be used simply as replacement fluids.** They can carry a similar risk of transmitting infections, such as HIV and hepatitis, as whole blood. They are also generally more expensive than crystalloid or synthetic colloid fluids.

See pp. 29–30 and 32.

# Synthetic colloid solutions

| GELATINS (Haemaccel, Gelofusine) | |
|---|---|
| Infection risk | None known at present |
| Indications | Replacement of blood volume |
| Precautions | <ul><li>May precipitate heart failure</li><li>Caution in renal insufficiency</li><li>Do not mix Haemaccel with citrated blood because of its high calcium concentration</li></ul> |
| Contraindications | Do not use in patients with established renal failure |
| Side-effects | <ul><li>Minor allergic reactions due to histamine release</li><li>Transient increase in bleeding time may occur</li><li>Hypersensitivity reactions may occur including, rarely, severe anaphylactic reactions</li></ul> |
| Dosage | No known dose limit |

## DEXTRAN 60 and DEXTRAN 70

| | |
|---|---|
| Infection risk | Nil |
| Indications | ■ Replacement of blood volume<br>■ Prophylaxis of postoperative venous thrombosis |
| Precautions | ■ Coagulation defects may occur<br>■ Platelet aggregation inhibited<br>■ Some preparations may interfere with compatibility testing of blood |
| Contraindications | Do not use in patients with pre-existing disorders of haemostasis and coagulation |
| Side-effects | ■ Minor allergic reactions<br>■ Transient increase in bleeding time may occur<br>■ Hypersensitivity reactions may occur including, rarely, severe anaphylactic reactions. Can be prevented with injection of 20 ml of Dextran 1 immediately before infusion, where available |
| Dosage | ■ Dextran 60: should not exceed 50 ml/kg body weight in 24 hours<br>■ Dextran 70: should not exceed 25 ml/kg body weight in 24 hours |

## DEXTRAN 40 and DEXTRAN 110

Not recommended as replacement fluids

## HYDROXYETHYL STARCH (Hetastarch or HES)

| | |
|---|---|
| Infection risk | Nil |
| Indications | Replacement of blood volume |
| Precautions | ■ Coagulation defects may occur |
| | ■ May precipitate volume overload and heart failure |
| Contraindications | ■ Do not use in patients with pre-existing disorders of haemostasis and coagulation |
| | ■ Do not use in patients with established renal failure |
| Side-effects | ■ Minor allergic reactions due to histamine release |
| | ■ Transient increase in bleeding time may occur |
| | ■ Hypersensitivity reactions may occur including, rarely, severe anaphylactic reactions |
| | ■ Serum amylase level may rise (not significant) |
| | ■ HES is retained in cells of the reticuloendothelial system; the long-term effects of this are unknown |
| Dosage | Should not usually exceed 20 ml/kg body weight in 24 hours |

**Notes**

# Blood products

## Key points

1  Safe blood products, used correctly, can be life-saving. However, even where quality standards are very high, transfusion carries some risks. If standards are poor or inconsistent, transfusion may be extremely risky.

2  No blood or blood product should be administered unless all nationally required tests have been carried out.

3  Each unit should be tested and labelled to show its ABO and RhD group.

4  Whole blood can be transfused to replace red cells in acute bleeding when there is also a need to correct hypovolaemia.

5  The preparation of blood components allows a single blood donation to provide treatment for two or three patients and also avoids the transfusion of elements of the whole blood that the patient may not require. Blood components can also be collected by apheresis.

6  Plasma can transmit most of the infections present in whole blood and there are very few indications for its transfusion.

7  Plasma derivatives are made by a pharmaceutical manufacturing process from large volumes of plasma comprising many individual blood donations. Plasma used in this process should be individually tested prior to pooling to minimize the risks of transmitting infection.

8  Factors VIII and IX and immunoglobulins are also made by recombinant DNA technology and are often favoured because there should be no risk of transmitting infectious agents to the patient. However, the costs are high and there have been some reported cases of complications.

| DEFINITIONS | |
|---|---|
| **Blood product** | Any therapeutic substance prepared from human blood |
| **Whole blood** | Unseparated blood collected into an approved container containing an anticoagulant-preservative solution |
| **Blood component** | 1  A constituent of blood, separated from whole blood, such as: <ul><li>Red cell concentrate</li><li>Red cell suspension</li><li>Plasma</li><li>Platelet concentrates</li></ul> 2  Plasma or platelets collected by apheresis [1]<br><br>3  Cryoprecipitate, prepared from fresh frozen plasma: rich in Factor VIII and fibrinogen |
| **Plasma derivative** [2] | Human plasma proteins prepared under pharmaceutical manufacturing conditions, such as: <ul><li>Albumin</li><li>Coagulation factor concentrates</li><li>Immunoglobulins</li></ul> |

**Note**

[1]  Apheresis: a method of collecting plasma or platelets directly from the donor, usually by a mechanical method

[2]  Processes for heat treatment or chemical treatment of plasma derivatives to reduce the risk of transmitting viruses are currently very effective against viruses that have lipid envelopes:

— HIV-1 and 2

— Hepatitis B and C

— HTLV-I and II

Inactivation of non-lipid-enveloped viruses such as hepatitis A and human parvovirus B19 is less effective

# Whole blood

## WHOLE BLOOD (CPD-Adenine-1)

A 450 ml whole blood donation contains:

| | |
|---|---|
| Description | Up to 510 ml total volume (volume may vary in accordance with local policies) |
| | ■ 450 ml donor blood |
| | ■ 63 ml anticoagulant-preservative solution |
| | ■ Haemoglobin approximately 12 g/ml |
| | ■ Haematocrit 35%–45% |
| | ■ No functional platelets |
| | ■ No labile coagulation factors (V and VIII) |
| Unit of issue | 1 donation, also referred to as a 'unit' or 'pack' |
| Infection risk | Not sterilized, so capable of transmitting any agent present in cells or plasma which has not been detected by routine screening for transfusion-transmissible infections, including HIV-1 and HIV-2, hepatitis B and C, other hepatitis viruses, syphilis, malaria and Chagas disease |
| Storage | ■ Between +2°C and +6°C in approved blood bank refrigerator, fitted with a temperature chart and alarm |
| | ■ During storage at +2°C and +6°C, changes in composition occur resulting from red cell metabolism |
| | ■ Transfusion should be started within 30 minutes of removal from refrigerator |
| Indications | ■ Red cell replacement in acute blood loss with hypovolaemia |
| | ■ Exchange transfusion |
| | ■ Patients needing red cell transfusions where red cell concentrates or suspensions are not available |
| Contraindications | Risk of volume overload in patients with: |
| | ■ Chronic anaemia |
| | ■ Incipient cardiac failure |
| Administration | ■ Must be ABO and RhD compatible with the recipient |
| | ■ Never add medication to a unit of blood |
| | ■ Complete transfusion within 4 hours of commencement |

## Blood components

### RED CELL CONCENTRATE ('Packed red cells', 'plasma-reduced blood'

| | |
|---|---|
| Description | ■ 150–200 ml red cells from which most of the plasma has been removed |
| | ■ Haemoglobin approximately 20 g/100 ml (not less than 45 g per unit) |
| | ■ Haematocrit 55%–75% |
| Unit of issue | 1 donation |
| Infection risk | Same as whole blood |
| Storage | Same as whole blood |
| Indications | ■ Replacement of red cells in anaemic patients |
| | ■ Use with crystalloid replacement fluids or colloid solution in acute blood loss |
| Administration | ■ Same as whole blood |
| | ■ To improve transfusion flow, normal saline (50–100 ml) may be added using a Y-pattern infusion set |

### RED CELL SUSPENSION

| | |
|---|---|
| Description | ■ 150–200 ml red cells with minimal residual plasma to which ±100 ml normal saline, adenine, glucose, mannitol solution (SAG-M) or an equivalent red cell nutrient solution has been added |
| | ■ Haemoglobin approximately 15 g/100 ml (not less than 45 g per unit) |
| | ■ Haematocrit 50%–70% |
| Unit of issue | 1 donation |
| Infection risk | Same as whole blood |
| Storage | Same as whole blood |
| Indications | Same as red cell concentrate |
| Contraindications | Not advised for exchange transfusion of neonates. The additive solution may be replaced with plasma, 45% albumin or an isotonic crystalloid solution, such as normal saline |
| Administration | ■ Same as whole blood |
| | ■ Better flow rates are achieved than with red cell concentrate or whole blood |

## LEUCOCYTE-DEPLETED RED CELLS

| | |
|---|---|
| Description | ■ A red cell suspension or concentrate containing $<5 \times 10^6$ white cells per pack, prepared by filtration through a leucocyte-depleting filter |
| | ■ Haemoglobin concentration and haematocrit depend on whether the product is whole blood, red cell concentrate or red cell suspension |
| | ■ Leucocyte depletion significantly reduces the risk of transmission of cytomegalovirus (CMV) |
| Unit of issue | 1 donation |
| Infection risk | Same as whole blood for all other transfusion-transmissible infections |
| Storage | Depends on production method: consult blood bank |
| Indications | ■ Minimizes white cell immunization in patients receiving repeated transfusions but, to achieve this, all blood components given to the patient must be leucocyte-depleted |
| | ■ Reduces risk of CMV transmission in special situations (see pp. 100 and 147) |
| | ■ Patients who have experienced two or more previous febrile reactions to red cell transfusion |
| Contraindications | Will not prevent graft-vs-host disease: for this purpose, blood components should be irradiated where facilities are available (radiation dose: 25–30 Gy) |
| Administration | ■ Same as whole blood |
| | ■ A leucocyte filter may also be used at the time of transfusion if leucocyte-depleted red cells or whole blood are not available |
| Alternative | ■ Buffy coat-removed whole blood or red cell suspension is usually effective in avoiding febrile non-haemolytic transfusion reactions |
| | ■ The blood bank should express the buffy coat in a sterile environment immediately before transporting the blood to the bedside |
| | ■ Start the transfusion within 30 minutes of delivery and use a leucocyte filter, where possible |
| | ■ Complete transfusion within 4 hours of commencement |

## PLATELET CONCENTRATES (prepared from whole blood donations)

| | |
|---|---|
| Description | Single donor unit in a volume of 50–60 ml of plasma should contain: |
| | ■ At least $55 \times 10^9$ platelets |
| | ■ $<1.2 \times 10^9$ red cells |
| | ■ $<0.12 \times 10^9$ leucocytes |
| Unit of issue | May be supplied as either: |
| | ■ Single donor unit: platelets prepared from one donation |
| | ■ Pooled unit: platelets prepared from 4 to 6 donor units 'pooled' into one pack to contain an adult dose of at least $240 \times 10^9$ platelets |
| Infection risk | ■ Same as whole blood, but a normal adult dose involves between 4 and 6 donor exposures |
| | ■ Bacterial contamination affects about 1% of pooled units |
| Storage | ■ Up to 72 hours at 20°C to 24°C (with agitation) unless collected in specialized platelet packs validated for longer storage periods; do not store at 2°C to 6°C |
| | ■ Longer storage increases the risk of bacterial proliferation and septicaemia in the recipient |
| Indications | ■ Treatment of bleeding due to: |
| | — Thrombocytopenia |
| | — Platelet function defects |
| | ■ Prevention of bleeding due to thrombocytopenia, such as in bone marrow failure |
| Contraindications | ■ Not generally indicated for prophylaxis of bleeding in surgical patients, unless known to have significant pre-operative platelet deficiency |
| | ■ Not indicated in: |
| | — Idiopathic autoimmune thrombocytopenic purpura (ITP) |
| | — Thrombotic thrombocytopenic purpura (TTP) |
| | — Untreated disseminated intravascular coagulation (DIC) |
| | — Thrombocytopenia associated with septicaemia, until treatment has commenced or in cases of hypersplenism |

| | |
|---|---|
| Dosage | ■ 1 unit of platelet concentrate/10 kg body weight: in a 60 or 70 kg adult, 4–6 single donor units containing at least 240 x $10^9$ platelets should raise the platelet count by 20–40 x $10^9$/L |
| | ■ Increment will be less if there is:<br>— Splenomegaly<br>— Disseminated intravascular coagulation<br>— Septicaemia |
| Administration | ■ After pooling, platelet concentrates should be infused as soon as possible, generally within 4 hours, because of the risk of bacterial proliferation |
| | ■ Must not be refrigerated before infusion as this reduces platelet function |
| | ■ 4–6 units of platelet concentrates (which may be supplied pooled) should be infused through a fresh standard blood administration set |
| | ■ Special platelet infusion sets are not required |
| | ■ Should be infused over a period of about 30 minutes |
| | ■ Do not give platelet concentrates prepared from RhD positive donors to an RhD negative female with child-bearing potential |
| | ■ Give platelet concentrates that are ABO compatible, whenever possible |
| Complications | Febrile non-haemolytic and allergic urticarial reactions are not uncommon, especially in patients receiving multiple transfusions (for management, see pp. 62–63) |

## PLATELET CONCENTRATES (collected by plateletpheresis)

| | |
|---|---|
| Description | ■ Volume 150–300 ml<br>■ Platelet content 150–500 x $10^9$, equivalent to 3–10 single donations<br>■ Platelet content, volume of plasma and leucocyte contamination depend on the collection procedure |
| Unit of issue | 1 pack containing platelet concentrates collected by a cell separator device from a single donor |
| Infection risk | Same as whole blood |
| Storage | Up to 72 hours at 20°C to 24°C (with agitation) unless collected in specialized platelet packs validated for longer storage periods; do not store at 2°C to 6°C |
| Indications | ■ Generally equivalent to the same dose of platelet concentrates prepared from whole blood<br>■ If a specially typed, compatible donor is required for the patient, several doses may be obtained from the selected donor |
| Dosage | 1 pack of platelet concentrate collected from a single donor by apheresis is usually equivalent to 1 therapeutic dose |
| Administration | Same as recovered donor platelets, but ABO compatibility is more important: high titre anti-A or anti-B in the donor plasma used to suspend the platelets may cause haemolysis of the recipient's red cells |

## FRESH FROZEN PLASMA

| | |
|---|---|
| Description | ■ Pack containing the plasma separated from one whole blood donation within 6 hours of collection and then rapidly frozen to –25°C or colder |
| | ■ Contains normal plasma levels of stable clotting factors, albumin and immunoglobulin |
| | ■ Factor VIII level at least 70% of normal fresh plasma level |
| Unit of issue | ■ Usual volume of pack is 200–300 ml |
| | ■ Smaller volume packs may be available for children |
| Infection risk | ■ If untreated, same as whole blood |
| | ■ Very low risk if treated with methylene blue/ultraviolet light inactivation (see virus 'inactivated' plasma) |
| Storage | ■ At –25°C or colder for up to 1 year |
| | ■ Before use, should be thawed in the blood bank in water which is between 30°C to 37°C. Higher temperatures will destroy clotting factors and proteins |
| | ■ Once thawed, should be stored in a refrigerator at +2°C to +6°C |
| Indications | ■ Replacement of multiple coagulation factor deficiencies: e.g. |
| | — Liver disease |
| | — Warfarin (anticoagulant) overdose |
| | — Depletion of coagulation factors in patients receiving large volume transfusions |
| | ■ Disseminated intravascular coagulation (DIC) |
| | ■ Thrombotic thrombocytopenic purpura (TTP) |
| Precautions | ■ Acute allergic reactions are not uncommon, especially with rapid infusions |
| | ■ Severe life-threatening anaphylactic reactions occasionally occur |
| | ■ Hypovolaemia alone is *not* an indication for use |
| Dosage | Initial dose of 15 ml/kg |

| Administration | ■ Must normally be ABO compatible to avoid risk of haemolysis in recipient |
| --- | --- |
| | ■ No compatibility testing required |
| | ■ Infuse using a standard blood administration set as soon as possible after thawing |
| | ■ Labile coagulation factors rapidly degrade; use within 6 hours of thawing |

## LIQUID PLASMA

| Description | ■ Plasma separated from a whole blood unit and stored at +4°C |
| --- | --- |
| | ■ No labile coagulation factors (Factors V and VIII) |

## FREEZE-DRIED POOLED PLASMA

| Description | ■ Plasma from many donors pooled before freeze-drying |
| --- | --- |
| Infection risk | ■ No virus inactivation step so the risk of transmitting infection is therefore multiplied many times |
| | ■ **This is an obsolete product that should not be used** |

## CRYOPRECIPITATE-DEPLETED PLASMA

| Description | Plasma from which approximately half the fibrinogen and Factor VIII has been removed as cryoprecipitate, but which contains all the other plasma constituents |
| --- | --- |

## VIRUS 'INACTIVATED' PLASMA

| Description | ■ Plasma treated with methylene blue/ultraviolet light inactivation to reduce the risk of HIV, hepatitis B and hepatitis C |
| --- | --- |
| | ■ The cost of this product is considerably higher than conventional fresh frozen plasma |
| Infection risk | The 'inactivation' of other viruses, such as hepatitis A and human parvovirus B19 is less effective |

## CRYOPRECIPITATE

| | |
|---|---|
| Description | ■ Prepared from fresh frozen plasma by collecting the precipitate formed during controlled thawing at +4°C and resuspending it in 10–20 ml plasma |
| | ■ Contains about half of the Factor VIII and fibrinogen in the donated whole blood: e.g. Factor VIII: 80–100 iu/pack; fibrinogen: 150–300 mg/pack |
| Unit of issue | Usually supplied as a single donor pack or a pack of 6 or more single donor units that have been pooled |
| Infection risk | As for plasma, but a normal adult dose involves at least 6 donor exposures |
| Storage | ■ At –25°C or colder for up to 1 year |
| Indications | ■ As an alternative to Factor VIII concentrate in the treatment of inherited deficiencies of: |
| | — von Willebrand Factor (von Willebrand's disease) |
| | — Factor VIII (haemophilia A) |
| | — Factor XIII |
| | ■ As a source of fibrinogen in acquired coagulopathies: e.g. disseminated intravascular coagulation (DIC) |
| Administration | ■ If possible, use ABO-compatible product |
| | ■ No compatibility testing required |
| | ■ After thawing, infuse as soon as possible through a standard blood administration set |
| | ■ Must be infused within 6 hours of thawing |

# Plasma derivatives

## HUMAN ALBUMIN SOLUTIONS

| | |
|---|---|
| Description | Prepared by fractionation of large pools of donated plasma |
| Preparations | ■ Albumin 5%: contains 50 mg/ml of albumin |
| | ■ Albumin 20%: contains 200 mg/ml of albumin |
| | ■ Albumin 25%: contains 250 mg/ml of albumin |
| | ■ Stable plasma protein solution (SPPS) and plasma protein fraction (PPF): similar albumin content to albumin 5% |
| Infection risk | No risk of transmission of viral infections if correctly manufactured |
| Indications | ■ Replacement fluid in therapeutic plasma exchange: use albumin 5% |
| | ■ Treatment of diuretic-resistant oedema in hypoproteinaemic patients: e.g. nephrotic syndrome or ascites. Use albumin 20% with a diuretic |
| | ■ Although 5% human albumin is currently licensed for a wide range of indications (e.g. volume replacement, burns and hypoalbuminaemia), there is *no* evidence that it is superior to saline solution or other crystalloid replacement fluids for acute plasma volume replacement |
| Precautions | Administration of 20% albumin may cause acute expansion of intravascular volume with risk of pulmonary oedema |
| Contraindications | Do not use for IV nutrition: it is an expensive and inefficient source of essential amino acids |
| Administration | ■ No compatibility testing required |
| | ■ No filter needed |

## COAGULATION FACTORS

### Factor VIII concentrate

| | |
|---|---|
| Description | ■ Partially purified Factor VIII prepared from large pools of donor plasma |
| | ■ Factor VIII ranges from 0.5–20 iu/mg of protein. Preparations with a higher activity are available |
| | ■ Products that are licensed in certain countries (e.g. USA and European Union) are all heated and/or chemically treated to reduce the risk of transmission of viruses |
| Unit of issue | Vials of freeze-dried protein labelled with content, usually about 250 iu of Factor VIII |
| Infection risk | Current virus 'inactivated' products do not appear to transmit HIV, HTLV, hepatitis C and other viruses that have lipid envelopes: the inactivation of non-enveloped viruses such as hepatitis A and parvovirus is less effective |
| Storage | +2°C to +6°C up to stated expiry date, unless otherwise indicated in manufacturer's instructions |
| Indications | ■ Treatment of haemophilia A |
| | ■ Treatment of von Willebrand's disease: use only preparations that contain von Willebrand Factor |
| Dosage | See p. 113 |
| Administration | ■ Reconstitute according to manufacturer's instructions |
| | ■ Once the powder is dissolved, draw up the solution using a filter needle and infuse through a standard infusion set within 2 hours |
| Alternatives | ■ Cryoprecipitate, fresh frozen plasma |
| | ■ Factor VIII prepared *in vitro* using recombinant DNA methods is commercially available. It is clinically equivalent to Factor VIII derived from plasma and does not have the risk of transmitting pathogens derived from plasma donors |

## PLASMA DERIVATIVES CONTAINING FACTOR IX

**Prothrombin complex concentrate (PCC)**
**Factor IX concentrate**

| Description | Contains: | PCC | Factor IX |
|---|---|---|---|
| | ■ Factors II, IX and X | ✔ | ✔ |
| | ■ Factor IX only | | ✔ |
| | ■ Some preparations also contain Factor VII | ✔ | |

| Unit of issue | Vials of freeze-dried protein labelled with content, usually about 350–600 iu of Factor IX |
|---|---|
| Infection risk | As Factor VIII |
| Storage | As Factor VIII |

| Indications | | PCC | Factor IX |
|---|---|---|---|
| | ■ Treatment of haemophilia B (Christmas disease) | ✔ | ✔ |
| | ■ Immediate correction of prolonged prothrombin time | ✔ | |

| Contraindications | PCC is not advised in patients with liver disease or thrombotic tendency |
|---|---|
| Dosage | See p. 114 |
| Administration | As Factor VIII |
| Alternatives | Plasma |

Factor IX produced *in vitro* by recombinant DNA methods will soon be available for the treatment of haemophilia B

## COAGULATION FACTOR PRODUCTS FOR PATIENTS WITH FACTOR VIII INHIBITORS

| Description | A heat-treated plasma fraction containing partly-activated coagulation factors |
|---|---|
| Infection risk | Probably the same as other heat-treated factor concentrates |
| Indications | Only for use in patients with inhibitors to Factor VIII |
| Administration | Should be used only with specialist advice |

## IMMUNOGLOBULINS

### Immunoglobulin for intramuscular use

| | |
|---|---|
| Description | Concentrated solution of the IgG antibody component of plasma |
| Preparations | Standard or normal immunoglobulin: prepared from large pools of donations and contains antibodies against infectious agents to which the donor population has been exposed |
| Infection risk | Transmission of virus infections has *not* been reported with intramuscular immunoglobulin |
| Indications | ■ Hyperimmune or specific immunoglobulin: from patients with high levels of specific antibodies to infectious agents: e.g. hepatitis B, rabies, tetanus<br>■ Prevention of specific infections<br>■ Treatment of immune deficiency states |
| Administration | Do not give intravenously as severe reactions occur |

### Anti-RhD immunoglobulin (Anti-D RhIG)

| | |
|---|---|
| Description | Prepared from plasma containing high levels of anti-RhD antibody from previously immunized persons |
| Indications | Prevention of haemolytic disease of the newborn in RhD-negative mothers (see pp. 132–134) |

### Immunoglobulin for intravenous use

| | |
|---|---|
| Description | As for intramuscular preparation, but with subsequent processing to render product safe for IV administration |
| Indications | ■ Idiopathic autoimmune thrombocytopenic purpura and some other immune disorders<br>■ Treatment of immune deficiency states<br>■ Hypogammaglobulinaemia<br>■ HIV-related disease |

# Notes

# Clinical transfusion procedures

## Key points

1 Every hospital should have standard operating procedures for each stage of the clinical transfusion process. All staff should be trained to follow them.

2 Clear communication and cooperation between clinical and blood bank staff are essential in ensuring the safety of blood issued for transfusion.

3 The blood bank should not issue blood for transfusion unless a blood sample label and blood request form have been correctly completed. The blood request form should include the reason for transfusion so that the most suitable product can be selected for compatibility testing.

4 Blood products should be kept within the correct storage conditions during transportation and in the clinical area before transfusion, in order to prevent loss of function or bacterial contamination.

5 The transfusion of an incompatible blood component is the most common cause of acute transfusion reactions, which may be fatal. The safe administration of blood depends on:
- Accurate, unique identification of the patient
- Correct labelling of the blood sample for pre-transfusion testing
- A final identity check of the patient and the blood unit to ensure the administration of the right blood to the right patient.

6 For each unit of blood transfused, the patient should be monitored by a trained member of staff before, during and on completion of the transfusion.

# Getting the right blood to the right patient at the right time

Once the decision to transfuse has been made, everyone involved in the clinical transfusion process has the responsibility to ensure the right blood gets to the right patient at the right time.

National guidelines on the clinical use of blood should always be followed in all hospitals where transfusions take place. If no national guidelines exist, each hospital should develop local guidelines and, ideally, establish a hospital transfusion committee to monitor clinical blood use and investigate any acute and delayed transfusion reactions.

Each hospital should ensure that the following are in place.

1 A blood request form.

2 A blood ordering schedule for common surgical procedures.

3 Guidelines on clinical and laboratory indications for the use of blood, blood products and simple alternatives to transfusion, including intravenous replacement fluids, and pharmaceuticals and medical devices to minimize the need for transfusion.

4 Standard operating procedures for each stage in the clinical transfusion process, including:
   - Ordering blood and blood products for elective/planned surgery
   - Ordering blood and blood products in an emergency
   - Completing the blood request form
   - Taking and labelling the pre-transfusion blood sample
   - Collecting blood and blood products from the blood bank
   - Storing and transporting blood and blood products, including storage in the clinical area
   - Administering blood and blood products, including the final patient identity check
   - Recording transfusions in patient records
   - Monitoring the patient before, during and after transfusion
   - Managing, investigating and recording transfusion reactions.

5 The training of all staff involved in the transfusion process to follow standard operating procedures.

The safety of the patient requiring transfusion depends on cooperation and effective communication between clinical and blood bank staff.

## GETTING THE RIGHT BLOOD TO THE RIGHT PATIENT AT THE RIGHT TIME

1   Assess the patient's clinical need for blood and when it is required.

2   Inform the patient and/or relatives about the proposed transfusion treatment and record in the patient's notes that you have done so.

3   Record the indications for transfusion in the patient's notes.

4   Select the blood product and quantity required. Use a blood ordering schedule as a guide to transfusion requirements for common surgical procedures.

5   Complete the blood request form accurately and legibly. Write the reason for transfusion so the blood bank can select the most suitable product for compatibility testing.

6   If blood is needed urgently, contact the blood bank by telephone immediately.

7   Obtain and correctly label a blood sample for compatibility testing.

8   Send the blood request form and blood sample to the blood bank.

9   Laboratory performs pre-transfusion antibody screening and compatibility tests and selects compatible units.

10  Delivery of blood products by blood bank or collection by clinical staff.

11  Store blood products in correct storage conditions if not immediately required for transfusion.

12  Check the identity on:
   ■ Patient
   ■ Blood product
   ■ Patient's documentation.

13  Administer the blood product.

14  Record in the patient's notes:
   ■ Type and volume of each product transfused
   ■ Unique donation number of each unit transfused
   ■ Blood group of each unit transfused
   ■ Time at which the transfusion of each unit commenced
   ■ Signature of the person administering the blood.

15  Monitor the patient before, during and on completion of the transfusion.

16  Record the completion of the transfusion.

17  Identify and respond immediately to any adverse effect. Record any transfusion reactions in the patient's notes.

For every patient requiring transfusion, it is the responsibility of the clinician to:

1 Correctly complete a blood request form.

2 Collect the blood sample from the right patient in the right sample tube and correctly label the sample tube.

3 Order blood in advance, whenever possible.

4 Provide the blood bank with clear information on:
- The products and number of units required
- The reason for transfusion
- The urgency of the patient's requirement for transfusion
- When and where the blood is required
- Who will deliver or collect the blood.

5 Ensure the correct storage of blood and blood products in the clinical area before transfusion.

6 Formally check the identity of the patient, the product and the documentation at the patient's bedside before transfusion.

7 Discard, or return to the blood bank for safe disposal, a blood pack that has been at room temperature for more than 4 hours (or whatever time is locally specified) or a pack that has been opened or shows any signs of deterioration.

8 Correctly record transfusions in the patient's notes:
- Reason for transfusion
- Product and volume transfused
- Time of transfusion
- Monitoring of the patient before, during and after transfusion
- Any adverse events.

## Patient identity
- Each patient should be identified using an identity wristband or some other firmly-attached marker with a unique hospital reference number
- This number should always be used on the blood sample tube and blood request form to identify the patient.

## Informing the patient
Whenever possible, explain the proposed transfusion to the patient or relatives and record in the patient's notes that you have done so.

# Ordering blood

```
Assess patient's
need for transfusion
```

| **Emergency** Blood needed within 1 hour or less | **Definite need for blood** e.g. elective surgery | **Possible need for blood** e.g. obstetrics, elective surgery |
|---|---|---|
| Urgently request ABO and RhD compatible units. Blood bank may select group O | Request ABO and RhD compatible units to be available at stated time | Request group, antibody screen and hold |

## Ordering blood for elective surgery

The timing of requests for blood for elective surgery should comply with local rules and the quantity requested should be guided by the local blood ordering schedule.

### Blood ordering schedule

Each hospital should develop a blood ordering schedule, which is a guide to normal transfusion requirements for common surgical procedures. The blood ordering schedule should reflect the clinical team's usual use of blood for common procedures, depending on their complexity and expected blood loss, and the supply of blood, blood products and alternatives to transfusion that are available.

An example of a blood ordering schedule is given on pp. 172–173.

The availability and use of intravenous crystalloid and colloid solutions is essential in all hospitals carrying out obstetrics and surgery.

Many operations do not require transfusion but, if there is a chance of major bleeding, it is essential that blood should be available promptly. By using the group, antibody screen and hold procedure (see p. 48), blood can be made available quickly without the need to 'commit' units of blood for one patient and so make them unavailable for others in need.

## Ordering blood in an emergency

It is essential that the procedures for ordering blood in an emergency are clear and simple and that everyone knows and follows them.

### ORDERING BLOOD IN AN EMERGENCY

1  Insert an IV cannula. Use it to take the blood sample for compatibility testing, set up an IV infusion of normal saline or a balanced salt solution (e.g. Ringer's lactate or Hartmann's solution). Send the blood sample to the blood bank as quickly as possible.

2  Clearly label the blood sample tube and the blood request form. If the patient is unidentified, use some form of **emergency admission number**. Use the patient's name only if you are sure you have correct information.

3  If you have to send another request for blood for the same patient within a short period, use the same identifiers used on the first request form and blood sample so the blood bank staff know they are dealing with the same patient.

4  If there are several staff working with emergency cases, one person should take charge of ordering blood and communicating with the blood bank about the incident. This is especially important if several injured patients are involved at the same time.

5  Tell the blood bank how quickly the blood is needed for each patient. Communicate using words that have been previously agreed with the blood bank to explain how urgently blood is required.

6  Make sure that both you and the blood bank staff know:
   ■  Who is going to bring the blood to the patient
   ■  Where the patient will be: e.g. operating theatre, delivery room.

7  The blood bank may send group O (and possibly RhD negative) blood, especially if there is any risk of errors in patient identification. During an acute emergency, this may be the safest way to avoid a serious mismatched transfusion.

## The blood request form

When blood is required for transfusion, the prescribing clinician should complete and sign a blood request form that provides the information shown in the example on p. 43.

## EXAMPLE OF BLOOD REQUEST FORM

Hospital _____     Date of request _____

### Patient details

Family name _____     Date of birth _____ Gender _____

Given name _____     Ward _____

Hospital reference no. _____     Blood group (if known) ABO [_____]

Address _____          RhD [_____]

_____

_____

### History

Diagnosis _____          Antibodies              Yes/No _____

Reason for transfusion _____     Previous transfusions   Yes/No _____

Anaemia _____          Any reactions            Yes/No _____

Relevant medical history _____   Previous pregnancies    Yes/No _____

### Request

☐ Group, screen and hold serum     Whole blood [_____] units

☐ Provide product                   Red cells   [_____] units

Date required _____       Plasma      [_____] units

Time required _____       Platelets   [_____] units

Deliver to _____          Other       [_____] units

**Name of doctor** (print) _____   **Signature** _____

---

**All the details requested on the blood request form must be completed accurately and legibly. If blood is needed urgently, also contact the blood bank by telephone immediately.**

---

It is essential that any request for blood, and the patient's blood sample accompanying it, are clearly labelled to:

- Uniquely identify the patient
- Indicate the type and number of units of blood product required
- Indicate the time and place at which it is needed.

# Blood samples for compatibility testing

**It is vital that the patient's blood sample is placed in a sample tube that is correctly labelled and is uniquely identifiable with the patient.**

## TAKING BLOOD SAMPLES FOR COMPATIBILITY TESTING

1   If the patient is conscious at the time of taking the sample, ask him or her to identify themselves by given name, family name, date of birth and any other appropriate information.

2   Check the patient's name against:
    - Patient's identity wristband or label
    - Patient's medical notes
    - Completed blood request form.

3   If the patient is unconscious, ask a relative or a second member of staff to verify the patient's identity.

4   Take the blood sample into the type of sample tube required by the blood bank. For adults, this is usually 10 ml, with no anticoagulant.

5   Label the sample tube clearly and accurately with the following information at the patient's bedside at the time the blood sample is being taken:
    - Patient's given name and family name
    - Patient's date of birth
    - Patient's hospital reference number
    - Patient's ward
    - Date
    - Signature of person taking the sample.

    Ensure that the patient's name is spelt correctly. Do not label the sample tube before obtaining the specimen because of the risk of putting the patient's blood into the wrong tube.

6   If the patient needs further red cell transfusion, send a new blood sample for compatibility testing.

    This is particularly important if the patient has had a recent red cell transfusion that was completed more than 24 hours earlier. Antibodies to red cells may appear very rapidly as a result of the immunological stimulus given by the transfused donor red cells.

    A fresh blood sample is essential to ensure that the patient does not receive blood which is now incompatible.

It is vital that all the details on the blood sample tube label match those on the blood request form and are uniquely identifiable with the patient.

Any failure to follow correct procedures can lead to incompatible transfusions. Blood bank staff are acting correctly if they refuse to accept a request for compatibility testing when either the blood request form or the patient's blood sample are inadequately identified or the details do not match. If there is any discrepancy, they should request a new sample and request form.

# Red cell compatibility testing

It is essential that all blood is tested before transfusion in order to:

- Ensure that transfused red cells are compatible with antibodies in the recipient's plasma
- Avoid stimulating the production of new red cell antibodies in the recipient, particularly anti-RhD.

All pre-transfusion test procedures should provide the following information about both the units of blood and the patient:

- ABO group
- RhD type
- Presence of red cell antibodies that could cause haemolysis in the recipient.

## ABO blood group antigens and antibodies

The ABO blood groups are the most important in clinical transfusion practice. There are four main red cell types: O, A, B and AB.

All healthy normal adults of group A, group B and group O have antibodies in their plasma against the red cell types (antigens) that they have not inherited:

- Group A individuals have antibody to group B
- Group B individuals have antibody to group A
- Group O individuals have antibody to group A *and* group B
- Group AB individuals do not have antibody to group A *or* B.

These antibodies are usually of IgM and IgG class and are normally able to haemolyse (destroy) transfused red cells.

# ABO incompatibility: haemolytic reactions

Anti-A or anti-B recipient antibodies are almost always capable of causing rapid destruction (haemolysis) of incompatible transfused red cells as soon as they enter the circulation.

A red cell transfusion that is not tested for compatibility carries a high risk of causing an acute haemolytic reaction. Similarly, if blood is given to the wrong patient, it may be incompatible.

The exact risk depends on the mix of ABO groups in the population. Typically, at least one third of unmatched transfusions will be ABO incompatible and at least 10% of these will lead to severe or fatal reactions.

In some circumstances, it is also important that the donor's antibodies are compatible with the patient's red cells. It is not always essential, however, to give blood of the same ABO group.

## RED CELL COMPONENTS

In red cell transfusion, there must be ABO and RhD compatibility between the donor's red cells and the recipient's plasma.

1 Group O individuals can receive blood from group O donors only

2 Group A individuals can receive blood from group A and O donors

3 Group B individuals can receive blood from group B and O donors

4 Group AB individuals can receive blood from AB donors, and also from group A, B and O donors

**Note:** Red cell concentrates, from which the plasma has been removed, are preferable when non-group specific blood is being transfused.

## PLASMA AND COMPONENTS CONTAINING PLASMA

In plasma transfusion, group AB plasma can be given to a patient of any ABO group because it contains neither anti-A nor anti-B antibody.

1 Group AB plasma (no antibodies) can be given to any ABO group patients

2 Group A plasma (anti-B) can be given to group O and A patients

3 Group B plasma (anti-A) can be given to group O and B patients

4 Group O plasma (anti-A + anti-B) can be given to group O patients only

**Safe transfusion depends on avoiding incompatibility between the donor's red cells and antibodies in the patient's plasma.**

1 Severe acute haemolytic transfusion reactions are invariably caused by transfusing red cells that are incompatible with the patient's ABO type. These reactions can be fatal. They most often result from:
   ■ Errors in labelling the patient's blood sample
   ■ Errors when collecting the unit of blood for transfusion
   ■ Failure to carry out the final identity check of the patient and the blood pack before infusing the unit of blood.

2 In some disease states, anti-A and anti-B may be difficult to detect in laboratory tests.

3 Young infants have IgG blood group antibodies that are passed on from the mother through the placenta. After birth, the infant starts to produce its own blood group antibodies.

## RhD red cell antigens and antibodies

Red cells have many other antigens but, in contrast to the ABO system, individuals very rarely make antibodies against these other antigens, unless they have been exposed to them ('immunized') by previous transfusion or during pregnancy and childbirth.

The most important is the RhD antigen. A single unit of RhD positive red cells transfused to an RhD negative person will usually provoke production of anti-RhD antibody. This can cause:
   ■ Haemolytic disease of the newborn in a subsequent pregnancy
   ■ Rapid destruction of a later transfusion of RhD positive red cells.

## Other red cell antigens and antibodies

There are many other antigens on the human red cell, each of which can stimulate production of antibody if transfused into a susceptible recipient. These antigen systems include:
   ■ Rh system: Rh C, c, E, e
   ■ Kidd
   ■ Kell
   ■ Duffy
   ■ Lewis.

These antibodies can also cause severe reactions to transfusion.

# Pre-transfusion testing (compatibility testing)

A direct test of compatibility (crossmatch) is usually performed before blood is infused. This detects a reaction between:

- **Patient's** serum
- **Donor** red cells.

The laboratory performs:

- Patient's ABO and RhD type
- Direct compatibility test or crossmatch.

These procedures normally take about 1 hour to complete. Shortened procedures are possible, but may fail to detect some incompatibilities.

## Compatibility problems

1 If the patient's sample has a clinically significant red cell antibody, the laboratory may need more time and may require a further blood sample in order to select compatible blood.

Non-urgent transfusions and surgery that is likely to require transfusion should be delayed until suitable blood is found.

2 If transfusion is needed urgently, the blood bank and the doctor responsible for the patient must balance the risk of delaying for full compatibility testing against the risk of transfusing blood that may not be completely compatible.

## Group, antibody screen and hold procedure

1 The patient's ABO and RhD type are determined.

2 The patient's serum is tested for clinically significant red cell antibodies.

3 The patient's serum sample is frozen and stored in the laboratory at –20°C, usually for seven days.

4 If blood is required within this period, the sample is thawed and used to perform an urgent compatibility test.

5 The blood bank should ensure that blood can be provided quickly if it is needed.

Using this method:

- Blood can be issued in 15–30 minutes
- It is unnecessary to hold crossmatched units of blood as an 'insurance' for a patient who is unlikely to need them
- Will reduce the workload and minimize the wastage of blood.

# Collecting blood products prior to transfusion

A common cause of transfusion reactions is the transfusion of an incorrect unit of blood that was intended for a different patient. This is often due to mistakes when collecting blood from the blood bank.

## COLLECTING BLOOD PRODUCTS FROM THE BLOOD BANK

1 Bring written documentation to identify the patient.

2 Check that the following details on the compatibility label attached to the blood pack exactly match the details on the patient's documentation:
   - Patient's family name and given name
   - Patient's hospital reference number
   - Patient's ward, operating room or clinic
   - Patient's ABO and RhD group.

3 Fill in the information required in the blood collection register.

## Storing blood products prior to transfusion

**All blood bank refrigerators should be specifically designed for blood storage.**

Once issued by the blood bank, the transfusion of whole blood, red cells and thawed fresh frozen plasma should be commenced within 30 minutes of their removal from refrigeration.

If the transfusion cannot be started within this period, they must be stored in an approved blood refrigerator at a temperature of 2°C to 6°C.

The temperature inside every refrigerator used for blood storage in wards and operating rooms should be monitored and recorded daily to ensure that the temperature remains between 2°C and 6°C.

If the ward or operating room does not have a refrigerator that is appropriate for storing blood, the blood should not be released from the blood bank until immediately before transfusion.

All unused blood products should be returned to the blood bank so that their return and reissue or safe disposal can be recorded.

# Whole blood and red cells

- Should be issued from the blood bank in a cold box or insulated carrier which will keep the temperature between 2°C and 6°C if the ambient (room) temperature is greater than 25°C or there is a possibility that the blood will not be transfused immediately

- Should be stored in the ward or operating theatre refrigerator at 2°C to 6°C until required for transfusion

- The upper limit of 6°C is essential to minimize the growth of any bacterial contamination in the unit of blood

- The lower limit of 2°C is essential to prevent haemolysis, which can cause fatal bleeding problems or renal failure.

**Whole blood and red cells should be infused within 30 minutes of removal from refrigeration.**

# Platelet concentrates

- Should be issued from the blood bank in a cold box or insulated carrier that will keep the temperature at about 20°C to 24°C

- Platelet concentrates that are held at lower temperatures lose their blood clotting capability; they should **never** be placed in a refrigerator

- Platelet concentrates should be transfused as soon as possible.

# Fresh frozen plasma and cryoprecipitate

- Fresh frozen plasma should be stored in the blood bank at a temperature of −25°C or colder until it is thawed before transfusion

- It should be thawed in the blood bank in accordance with approved procedures and issued in a blood transport box in which the temperature is maintained between 2°C and 6°C

- Fresh frozen plasma should be infused within 30 minutes of thawing

- If not required for immediate use, it should be stored in a refrigerator at a temperature of 2°C to 6°C and transfused within 24 hours

- As with whole blood or red cells, bacteria can proliferate in plasma that is held at ambient (room) temperature

- Most of the coagulation factors are stable at refrigerator temperatures, except for Factor V and Factor VIII:
  — If plasma is not stored frozen at −25°C or colder, Factor VIII falls rapidly over 24 hours. Plasma with a reduced Factor VIII level is of no use for the treatment of haemophilia, although it can be used in other clotting problems
  — Factor V declines more slowly.

# Administering blood products

Every hospital should have written standard operating procedures for the administration of blood products, particularly for the final identity check of the patient, the blood pack, the compatibility label and the documentation.

For each unit of blood supplied, the blood bank should provide documentation stating:

- Patient's family name and given name
- Patient's ABO and RhD group
- Unique donation number of the blood pack
- Blood group of the blood pack.

## Compatibility label

A compatibility label should be attached firmly to each unit of blood, showing the following information.

---

**THIS BLOOD IS COMPATIBLE WITH:**          Blood pack no. [          ]

Patient's name:

Patient's hospital reference number or date of birth:

Patient's ward:

Patient's ABO and RhD group:

Expiry date:

Date of compatibility test:

Blood group of blood pack:

**RETURN BLOOD PROMPTLY TO BLOOD BANK IF NOT USED**

---

## Checking the blood pack

The blood pack should always be inspected for signs of deterioration:

- On arrival in the ward or operating room
- Before transfusion, if it is not used immediately.

**Discoloration or signs of any leakage may be the only warning that the blood has been contaminated by bacteria and could cause a severe or fatal reaction when transfused.**

Check for:

1  Any sign of haemolysis in the plasma indicating that the blood has been contaminated, allowed to freeze or become too warm.

2  Any sign of haemolysis on the line between the red cells and plasma.

3  Any sign of contamination, such as a change of colour in the red cells, which often look darker or purple/black when contaminated.

4  Any clots, which may mean that the blood was not mixed properly with the anticoagulant when it was collected or might also indicate bacterial contamination due to the utilization of citrate by proliferating bacteria.

5  Any signs that there is a leak in the pack or that it has already been opened.

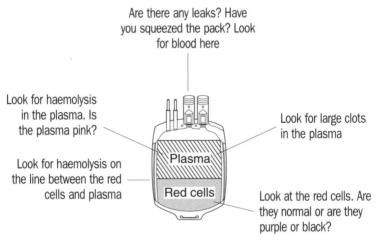

Are there any leaks? Have you squeezed the pack? Look for blood here

Look for haemolysis in the plasma. Is the plasma pink?

Look for large clots in the plasma

Plasma

Look for haemolysis on the line between the red cells and plasma

Red cells

Look at the red cells. Are they normal or are they purple or black?

**Do not administer the transfusion if the blood pack appears abnormal or damaged or it has been (or may have been) out of the refrigerator for longer than 30 minutes. Inform the blood bank immediately.**

## Checking the patient's identity and the blood pack before transfusion

Before starting the infusion, it is vital to make the final identity check in accordance with your hospital's standard operating procedure.

The final identity check should be undertaken **at the patient's bedside** immediately before commencing the administration of the blood product. It should be undertaken by two people, at least one of whom should be a registered nurse or doctor.

---

### THE FINAL PATIENT IDENTITY CHECK

1  Ask the patient to identify himself/herself by family name, given name, date of birth and any other appropriate information.

   If the patient is unconscious, ask a relative or a second member of staff to state the patient's identity.

2  Check the patient's identity and gender against:
   - Patient's identity wristband or label
   - Patient's medical notes.

3  Check that the following details on the compatibility label attached to the blood pack exactly match the details on the patient's documentation **and** identity wristband:
   - Patient's family name and given name
   - Patient's hospital reference number
   - Patient's ward or operating room
   - Patient's blood group.

4  Check that there are no discrepancies between the ABO and RhD group on:
   - Blood pack
   - Compatibility label.

5  Check that there are no discrepancies between the unique donation number on:
   - Blood pack
   - Compatibility label.

6  Check that the expiry date on the blood pack has not been passed.

The final check at the patient's bedside is the last opportunity to detect an identification error and prevent a potentially incompatible transfusion, which may be fatal.

## Time limits for infusion

There is a risk of bacterial proliferation or loss of function in blood products once they have been removed from the correct storage conditions.

| TIME LIMITS FOR INFUSION | | |
| --- | --- | --- |
| | **Start infusion** | **Complete infusion** |
| Whole blood or red cells | Within 30 minutes of removing pack from refrigerator | Within 4 hours (or less in high ambient temperature) |
| Platelet concentrates | Immediately | Within 20 minutes |
| Fresh frozen plasma and cryoprecipitate | As soon as possible | Within 20 minutes |

## Disposable equipment for blood administration
Cannulas for infusing blood products:
- Must be sterile and must **never** be reused
- Use flexible plastic cannulas, if possible, as they are safer and preserve the veins
- A doubling of the diameter of the cannula increases the flow rate of most fluids by a factor of 16.

### Whole blood, red cells, plasma and cryoprecipitate
- Use a new, sterile blood administration set containing an integral 170–200 micron filter
- Change the set at least 12-hourly during blood component infusion
- In a very warm climate, change the set more frequently and usually after every four units of blood, if given within a 12-hour period

### Platelet concentrates

Use a fresh blood administration set or platelet transfusion set, primed with saline.

### Paediatric patients

■ Use a special paediatric set for paediatric patients, if possible

■ These allow the blood or other infusion fluid to flow into a graduated container built into the infusion set

■ This permits the volume given, and the rate of infusion, to be controlled simply and accurately.

## Warming blood

There is no evidence that warming blood is beneficial to the patient when infusion is slow.

At infusion rates greater than 100 ml/minute, cold blood may be a contributing factor in cardiac arrest. However, keeping the patient warm is probably more important than warming the infused blood.

Warmed blood is most commonly required in:

■ Large volume rapid transfusions:

— Adults: greater than 50 ml/kg/hour

— Children: greater than 15 ml/kg/hour

■ Exchange transfusion in infants

■ Patients with clinically significant cold agglutinins.

Blood should only be warmed in a blood warmer. Blood warmers should have a visible thermometer and an audible warning alarm and should be properly maintained. Older types of blood warmer may slow the infusion rate of fluids.

**Blood should never be warmed in a bowl of hot water as this could lead to haemolysis of the red cells which could be life-threatening.**

## Pharmaceuticals and blood products

1 Do not add any medicines or any infusion solutions other than normal saline (sodium chloride 0.9%) to any blood component.

2 Use a separate IV line if an intravenous fluid other than normal saline has to be given at the same time as blood components.

# Recording the transfusion

Before administering blood products, it is important to write the reason for transfusion in the patient's case-notes. If the patient later has a problem that could be related to the transfusion, the records should show who ordered the products and why. This information is also useful for conducting an audit of transfusion practice.

The record you make in the patient's case-notes is your best protection if there is any medico-legal challenge later on.

---

## RECORDING THE TRANSFUSION

The following information should be recorded in the patient's notes.

1 Whether the patient and/or relatives have been informed about the proposed transfusion treatment.

2 The reason for transfusion.

3 Signature of the prescribing clinician.

4 Pre-transfusion checks of:
- Patient's identity
- Blood pack
- Compatibility label
- Signature of the person performing the pre-transfusion identity check.

5 The transfusion:
- Type and volume of each product transfused
- Unique donation number of each unit transfused
- Blood group of each unit transfused
- Time at which the transfusion of each unit commenced
- Signature of the person administering the blood component
- Monitoring of the patient before, during and after the transfusion.

6 Any transfusion reactions.

---

# Monitoring the transfused patient

It is essential to take baseline observations and to ensure that the patient is being monitored during and after the transfusion in order to detect any adverse event as early as possible. This will ensure that potentially life-saving action can be taken quickly.

Before commencing the transfusion, it is essential to:

- Encourage the patient to notify a nurse or doctor immediately if he or she becomes aware of any reactions such as shivering, flushing, pain or shortness of breath or begins to feel anxious

- Ensure that the patient is in a setting where he or she can be directly observed.

## MONITORING THE TRANSFUSED PATIENT

1  **For each unit of blood transfused**, monitor the patient:
   - Before starting the transfusion
   - As soon as the transfusion is started
   - 15 minutes after starting the transfusion
   - At least every hour during transfusion
   - On completion of the transfusion
   - 4 hours after completing the transfusion.

2  At each of these stages, record the following information on the patient's chart:
   - Patient's general appearance
   - Temperature
   - Pulse
   - Blood pressure
   - Respiratory rate
   - Fluid balance:
     — Oral and IV fluid intake
     — Urinary output.

3  Record:
   - Time the transfusion is started
   - Time the transfusion is completed
   - Volume and type of all products transfused
   - Unique donation numbers of all products transfused
   - Any adverse effects.

**Severe reactions most commonly present during the first 15 minutes of a transfusion. All patients and, in particular, unconscious patients should be monitored during this period and for the first 15 minutes of each subsequent unit.**

The transfusion of each unit of the blood or blood component should be completed within four hours of the pack being punctured. If a unit is not completed within four hours, discontinue its use and dispose of the remainder through the clinical waste system.

## Acute transfusion reactions

If the patient appears to be experiencing an adverse reaction, stop the transfusion and seek urgent medical assistance. Record vital signs regularly until the medical officer has assessed the patient.

See pp. 62–65 for the clinical features and management of acute transfusion reactions.

In the case of a suspected transfusion reaction, do not discard the blood pack and infusion set, but return them to the blood bank for investigation.

Record the clinical details and actions taken in the patient's case-notes.

# Notes

# Adverse effects of transfusion

## Key points

1  All suspected acute transfusion reactions should be reported immediately to the blood bank and to the doctor who is responsible for the patient. Seek assistance from experienced colleagues.

2  Acute reactions may occur in 1% to 2% of transfused patients. Rapid recognition and management of the reaction may save the patient's life. Once immediate action has been taken, careful and repeated clinical assessment is essential to identify and treat the patient's main problems.

3  Errors and failure to adhere to correct procedures are the commonest cause of life-threatening acute haemolytic transfusion reactions.

4  Bacterial contamination in red cells or platelet concentrates is an under-recognized cause of acute transfusion reactions.

5  Patients who receive regular transfusions are particularly at risk of acute febrile reactions. With experience, these can be recognized so that transfusions are not delayed or stopped unnecessarily.

6  Transfusion-transmitted infections are the most serious delayed complications of transfusion. Since a delayed transfusion reaction may occur days, weeks or months after the transfusion, the association with the transfusion may easily be missed. It is therefore essential to record all transfusions accurately in the patient's case notes and to consider transfusion in the differential diagnosis.

7  The infusion of large volumes of blood and intravenous fluids may cause haemostatic defects or metabolic disturbances.

# Acute complications of transfusion

Acute transfusion reactions occur during or shortly after (within 24 hours) the transfusion.

## Initial management and investigation

When an acute reaction first occurs, it may be difficult to decide on its type and severity as the signs and symptoms may not initially be specific or diagnostic. However, with the exception of allergic urticarial and febrile non-haemolytic reactions, all are potentially fatal and require urgent treatment.

**In an unconscious or anaesthetized patient, hypotension and uncontrolled bleeding may be the only signs of an incompatible transfusion.**

**In a conscious patient undergoing a severe haemolytic transfusion reaction, signs and symptoms may appear within minutes of infusing only 5–10 ml of blood. Close observation at the start of the infusion of each unit is essential.**

If an acute transfusion reaction occurs, first check the blood pack labels and the patient's identity. If there is any discrepancy, stop the transfusion immediately and consult the blood bank.

In order to rule out any possible identification errors in the clinical area or blood bank, stop all transfusions in the same ward or operating room until they have been carefully checked. In addition, request the blood bank to stop issuing any blood for transfusion until the cause of the reaction has been fully investigated and to check whether any other patient is receiving transfusion, especially in the same ward or operating room, or at the same time.

See pages 62–65 for the signs and symptoms, possible causes and management of the three broad categories of acute transfusion reaction to aid in immediate management.

Page 66 summarizes the drugs and dosages that may be needed in managing acute transfusion reactions.

# Guidelines for the recognition and management of acute transfusion reactions

## CATEGORY 1: MILD REACTIONS

| Signs | Symptoms | Possible cause |
|---|---|---|
| ■ Localized cutaneous reactions:<br> — Urticaria<br> — Rash | ■ Pruritus (itching) | ■ Hypersensitivity (mild) |

## CATEGORY 2: MODERATELY SEVERE REACTIONS

| Signs | Symptoms | Possible cause |
|---|---|---|
| ■ Flushing<br>■ Urticaria<br>■ Rigors<br>■ Fever<br>■ Restlessness<br>■ Tachycardia | ■ Anxiety<br>■ Pruritus<br>■ Palpitations<br>■ Mild dyspnoea<br>■ Headache | ■ Hypersensitivity (moderate–severe)<br>■ Febrile non-haemolytic transfusion reactions:<br> — Antibodies to white blood cells, platelets<br> — Antibodies to proteins, including IgA<br>■ Possible contamination with pyrogens and/or bacteria |

## CATEGORY 1: MILD REACTIONS

### Immediate management

1 Slow the transfusion.

2 Administer antihistamine IM (e.g. chlorpheniramine 0.1 mg/kg or equivalent).

3 If no clinical improvement within 30 minutes or if signs and symptoms worsen, **treat as Category 2**.

## CATEGORY 2: MODERATELY SEVERE REACTIONS

### Immediate management

1 Stop the transfusion. Replace the infusion set and keep IV line open with normal saline.

2 Notify the doctor responsible for the patient and the blood bank immediately.

3 Send blood unit with infusion set, freshly collected urine and new blood samples (1 clotted and 1 anticoagulated) from vein opposite infusion site with appropriate request form to blood bank for laboratory investigations.

4 Administer antihistamine IM (e.g. chlorpheniramine 0.1 mg/kg or equivalent) and oral or rectal antipyretic (e.g. paracetamol 10 mg/kg: 500 mg – 1 g in adults). Avoid aspirin in thrombocytopenic patients.

5 Give IV corticosteroids and bronchodilators if there are anaphylactoid features (e.g. broncospasm, stridor).

6 Collect urine for next 24 hours for evidence of haemolysis and send to laboratory.

7 If clinical improvement, restart transfusion slowly with new blood unit and observe carefully.

8 If no clinical improvement within 15 minutes or if signs and symptoms worsen, **treat as Category 3**.

## CATEGORY 3: LIFE-THREATENING REACTIONS

### Signs

- Rigors
- Fever
- Restlessness
- Hypotension (fall of 20% in systolic BP)
- Tachycardia (rise of 20% in heart rate)
- Haemoglobinuria (red urine)
- Unexplained bleeding (DIC)

### Symptoms

- Anxiety
- Chest pain
- Pain near infusion site
- Respiratory distress/ shortness of breath
- Loin/back pain
- Headache
- Dyspnoea

### Possible causes

- Acute intravascular haemolysis
- Bacterial contamination and septic shock
- Fluid overload
- Anaphylaxis
- Transfusion-associated acute lung injury (TRALI)

### Note

1   If an acute transfusion reaction occurs, first check the blood pack labels and the patient's identity. If there is any discrepancy, stop the transfusion immediately and consult the blood bank.

2   In an unconscious or anaesthetized patient, hypotension and uncontrolled bleeding may be the only signs of an incompatible transfusion.

3   In a conscious patient undergoing a severe haemolytic transfusion reaction, signs and symptoms may appear very quickly – within minutes of infusing only 5–10 ml of blood. Close observation at the start of the infusion of each unit is essential.

## CATEGORY 3: LIFE-THREATENING REACTIONS

### Immediate management

1 Stop the transfusion. Replace the infusion set and keep IV line open with normal saline.

2 Infuse normal saline (initially 20–30 ml/kg) to maintain systolic BP. If hypotensive, give over 5 minutes and elevate patient's legs.

3 Maintain airway and give high flow oxygen by mask.

4 Give adrenaline (as 1:1000 solution) 0.01 mg/kg body weight by slow intramuscular injection.

5 Give IV corticosteroids and bronchodilators if there are anaphylactoid features (e.g. broncospasm, stridor).

6 Give diuretic: e.g. frusemide 1 mg/kg IV or equivalent.

7 Notify the doctor responsible for patient and blood bank immediately.

8 Send blood unit with infusion set, fresh urine sample and new blood samples (1 clotted and 1 anticoagulated) from vein opposite infusion site with appropriate request form to blood bank for investigations.

9 Check a fresh urine specimen visually for signs of haemoglobinuria.

10 Start a 24-hour urine collection and fluid balance chart and record all intake and output. Maintain fluid balance.

11 Assess for bleeding from puncture sites or wounds. If there is clinical or laboratory evidence of DIC (see p. 115—117), give platelets (adult: 5–6 units) **and** either cryoprecipitate (adult: 12 units) *or* fresh frozen plasma (adult: 3 units).

12 Reassess. If hypotensive:
   ■ Give further saline 20–30 ml/kg over 5 minutes
   ■ Give inotrope, if available.

13 If urine output falling or laboratory evidence of acute renal failure (rising $K^+$, urea, creatinine):
   ■ Maintain fluid balance accurately
   ■ Give further frusemide
   ■ Consider dopamine infusion, if available
   ■ Seek expert help: the patient may need renal dialysis.

14 If bacteraemia is suspected (rigors, fever, collapse, no evidence of a haemolytic reaction), start broad-spectrum antibiotics IV.

| TYPE OF DRUG | EFFECTS | EXAMPLES | | NOTES |
|---|---|---|---|---|
| | | Name | Route/Dose | |
| Intravenous replacement fluid | Expands blood volume | Normal saline | If patient hypotensive, 20–30 ml/kg over 5 minutes | Avoid colloid solutions |
| Antipyretic | Reduces fever and inflammatory response | Paracetemol | Oral or rectal 10 mg/kg | Avoid aspirin-containing products if low platelet count |
| Antihistamine | Inhibits histamine mediated responses | Chlorphen-iramine | IM or IV 0.1 mg/kg | |
| Bronchodilator | Inhibits immune mediated bronchospasm | Adrenaline | 0.01 mg/kg (as 1: 1000 solution) by slow IM injection | Dose may be repeated every 10 minutes, according to BP and pulse until improvement |
| | | Consider salbutamol | By nebuliser | |
| | | Aminophylline | 5 mg/kg | |
| Inotrope | Increases myocardial contractility | Dopamine | IV infusion 1 $\mu$g/kg/minute | ■ Low doses induce vaso-dilation and improve renal perfusion |
| | | Dobutamine | IV infusion 1–10 $\mu$g/kg/minute | ■ Doses above 5 $\mu$g/kg/minute cause vaso-constriction and worsen heart failure |
| Diuretic | Inhibits fluid reabsorption from ascending loop of Henle | Frusemide | Slow IV injection 1 mg/kg | |

## INVESTIGATING ACUTE TRANSFUSION REACTIONS

1   Immediately report all acute transfusion reactions, with the exception of mild hypersensitivity (Category 1), to the doctor responsible for the patient and to the blood bank that supplied the blood.

   If you suspect a severe life-threatening reaction, seek help immediately from the duty anaesthetist, emergency team or whoever is available and skilled to assist.

2   Record the following information on the patient's notes:
   - Type of transfusion reaction
   - Length of time after the start of transfusion that the reaction occurred
   - Volume, type and pack numbers of the blood products transfused.

3   Take the following samples and send them to the blood bank for laboratory investigations:
   - Immediate post-transfusion blood samples (1 clotted and 1 anticoagulated: EDTA/Sequestrene) from the vein opposite the infusion site for:
     — Repeat ABO and RhD group
     — Repeat antibody screen and crossmatch
     — Full blood count
     — Coagulation screen
     — Direct antiglobulin test
     — Urea and creatinine
     — Electrolytes
   - Blood culture in a special blood culture bottle
   - Blood unit and infusion set containing red cell and plasma residues from the transfused donor blood
   - First specimen of the patient's urine following the reaction.

4   Complete a transfusion reaction report form.

5   After the initial investigation of the reaction, send the following to the blood bank for laboratory investigations:
   - Blood samples (1 clotted and 1 anticoagulated: EDTA/Sequestrene) taken from the vein opposite the infusion site 12 hours and 24 hours after the start of the reaction
   - Patient's 24-hour urine sample.

6   Record the results of the investigations in the patient's records for future follow-up, if required.

## Acute intravascular haemolysis

1  Acute intravascular haemolytic reactions are caused by the infusion of incompatible red cells. Antibodies in the patient's plasma haemolyse the incompatible transfused red cells.

2  Even a small volume (10–50 ml) of incompatible blood can cause a severe reaction and larger volumes increase the risk.

3  The most common cause is an ABO incompatible transfusion. This almost always arises from:
   ■  Errors in the blood request form
   ■  Taking blood from the wrong patient into a pre-labelled sample tube
   ■  Incorrect labelling of the blood sample tube sent to the blood bank
   ■  Inadequate checks of the blood against the identity of the patient before starting a transfusion.

4  Antibodies in the patient's plasma against other blood group antigens of the transfused blood, such as Kidd, Kell or Duffy systems, can also cause acute intravascular haemolysis.

5  In the conscious patient, signs and symptoms usually appear within minutes of commencing the transfusion, sometimes when less than 10 ml have been given.

6  In an unconscious or anaesthetized patient, hypotension and uncontrollable bleeding due to disseminated intravascular coagulation (DIC) may be the only signs of an incompatible transfusion.

7  It is therefore essential to monitor the patient at the start of the transfusion of **each** unit of blood.

### Prevention

1  Correctly label blood samples and request forms.

2  Place the patient's blood sample in the correct sample tube.

3  Always check the blood against the identity of the patient at the bedside before transfusion.

## Bacterial contamination and septic shock

1  Bacterial contamination affects up to 0.4% of red cells and 1–2% of platelet concentrates.

2  Blood may become contaminated by:
   ■ Bacteria from the donor's skin during blood collection (usually skin *staphylococci*)
   ■ A bacteraemia present in the blood of a donor at the time the blood is collected (e.g. *Yersinia*)
   ■ Improper handling in blood processing
   ■ Defects or damage to the plastic blood pack
   ■ Thawing fresh frozen plasma or cryoprecipitate in a water-bath (often contaminated).

3  Some contaminants, particularly *Pseudomonas* species, grow at 2°C to 6°C and so can survive or multiply in refrigerated red cell units. The risk therefore increases with the time out of refrigeration.

4  *Staphylococci* grow in warmer conditions and proliferate in platelet concentrates at 20°C to 24°C, limiting their storage life.

5  Signs usually appear rapidly after starting infusion, but may be delayed for a few hours.

6  A severe reaction may be characterized by sudden onset of high fever, rigors and hypotension.

7  Urgent supportive care and high-dose intravenous antibiotics are required.

## Fluid overload

1  Fluid overload can result in heart failure and pulmonary oedema.

2  May occur when:
   ■ Too much fluid is transfused
   ■ The transfusion is too rapid
   ■ Renal function is impaired.

3  Fluid overload is particularly likely to happen in patients with:
   ■ Chronic severe anaemia
   ■ Underlying cardiovascular disease.

## Anaphylactic reaction

1  A rare complication of transfusion of blood components or plasma derivatives.

2   The risk is increased by rapid infusion, typically when fresh frozen plasma is used as an exchange fluid in therapeutic plasma exchange.

3   Cytokines in the plasma may be one cause of broncho-constriction and vasoconstriction in occasional recipients.

4   IgA deficiency in the recipient is a rare cause of very severe anaphylaxis. This can be caused by any blood product since most contain traces of IgA.

5   Occurs within minutes of starting the transfusion and is characterized by:
   ■ Cardiovascular collapse
   ■ Respiratory distress
   ■ No fever.

6   Anaphylaxis is likely to be fatal if it is not managed rapidly and aggressively.

## Transfusion-associated acute lung injury (TRALI)

1   Usually caused by donor plasma that contains antibodies against the patient's leucocytes.

2   Rapid failure of pulmonary function usually presents within 1 to 4 hours of starting transfusion, with diffuse opacity on the chest X-ray.

3   There is no specific therapy. Intensive respiratory and general support in an intensive care unit is required.

## Delayed complications of transfusion

### Delayed haemolytic transfusion reactions

#### Signs and symptoms

1   Signs appear 5–10 days after transfusion:
   ■ Fever
   ■ Anaemia
   ■ Jaundice
   ■ Occasionally haemoglobinuria.

2   Severe, life-threatening delayed haemolytic transfusion reactions with shock, renal failure and DIC are rare.

| COMPLICATION | PRESENTATION | TREATMENT |
|---|---|---|
| Delayed haemolytic reactions | 5–10 days post-transfusion:<br>■ Fever<br>■ Anaemia<br>■ Jaundice | ■ Usually no treatment<br>■ If hypotension and oliguria, treat as acute intravascular haemolysis |
| Post-transfusion purpura | 5–10 days post-transfusion:<br>■ Increased bleeding tendency<br>■ Thrombocytopenia | ■ High dose steroids<br>■ High dose intravenous immunoglobulin<br>■ Plasma exchange |
| Graft-vs-host disease | 10–12 days post-transfusion:<br>■ Fever<br>■ Skin rash and desquamation<br>■ Diarrhoea<br>■ Hepatitis<br>■ Pancytopenia | ■ Usually fatal<br>■ Supportive care<br>■ No specific therapy |
| Iron overload | Cardiac and liver failure in transfusion-dependent patients | ■ Prevent with iron-binding agents: e.g. desferrioxamine |

## Management

1 No treatment is normally required.

2 Treat as for acute intravascular haemolysis if hypotension and renal failure occur.

3 Investigations:
   ■ Recheck the patient's blood group
   ■ Direct antiglobulin test is usually positive
   ■ Raised unconjugated bilirubin.

### Prevention

1 Careful laboratory screening for red cell antibodies in the patient's plasma and the selection of red cells compatible with these antibodies.

2 Some reactions are due to rare antigens (i.e. anti-$Jk^a$ blood group antibodies that are difficult to detect pre-transfusion).

## Post-transfusion purpura

1 A rare but potentially fatal complication of transfusion of red cells or platelet concentrates, caused by antibodies directed against platelet-specific antigens in the recipient.

2 Most commonly seen in female patients.

### Signs and symptoms

- Signs of bleeding
- Acute, severe thrombocytopenia 5–10 days after transfusion, defined as a platelet count of less than 100 x $10^9$/L.

### Management

Management becomes clinically important at a platelet count of 50 x $10^9$/L, with a danger of hidden occult bleeding at 20 x $10^9$/L.

1 Give high dose corticosteroids.

2 Give high dose IV immunoglobulin, 2 g/kg or 0.4 g/kg for 5 days.

3 Plasma exchange.

4 Monitor the patient's platelet count: normal range is 150 x $10^9$/L – 440 x $10^9$/L.

5 It is preferable to give platelet concentrates of the same ABO type as the patient's.

6 If available, give platelet concentrates that are negative for the platelet-specific antigen against which the antibodies are directed.

7 Unmatched platelet transfusion is generally ineffective. Recovery of platelet count after 2–4 weeks is usual.

### Prevention

Expert advice is essential and only platelet concentrates that are compatible with the patient's antibodies should be used.

# Graft-versus-host disease

1   A rare and potentially fatal complication of transfusion.

2   Occurs in such patients as:
    ■ Immunodeficient recipients of bone marrow transplants
    ■ Immunocompetent patients transfused with blood from individuals with whom they have a compatible tissue type (HLA: human leucocyte antigen), usually blood relatives.

## Signs and symptoms

1   Typically occurs 10–12 days after transfusion.

2   Characterized by:
    ■ Fever
    ■ Skin rash and desquamation
    ■ Diarrhoea
    ■ Hepatitis
    ■ Pancytopenia.

## Management

Usually fatal. Treatment is supportive; there is no specific therapy.

## Prevention

Gamma irradiation of cellular blood components to stop the proliferation of transfused lymphocytes.

# Iron overload

There are no physiological mechanisms to eliminate excess iron and thus transfusion-dependent patients can, over a long period of time, accumulate iron in the body resulting in haemosiderosis.

## Signs and symptoms

Organ failure, particularly of the heart and liver in transfusion-dependent patients.

## Management and prevention

1   Iron-binding agents, such as desferrioxamine, are widely used to minimize the accumulation of iron in transfusion-dependent patients (see pp. 107–108).

2   Aim to keep serum ferritin levels at <2000 mg/litre.

## Delayed complications of transfusion: transfusion-transmitted infections

The following infections may be transmitted by transfusion:

- HIV-1 and HIV-2
- HTLV-I and HTLV-II
- Hepatitis B and C
- Syphilis (*Treponema pallidum*)
- Chagas disease (*Trypanosoma cruzi*)
- Malaria
- Cytomegalovirus (CMV)
- Other rare transfusion-transmissible infections, including human parvovirus B19, brucellosis, Epstein-Barr virus, toxoplasmosis, infectious mononucleosis and Lymes' disease.

Since a delayed transfusion reaction may occur days, weeks or months after the transfusion, the association with the transfusion may easily be missed.

It is essential to record all transfusions accurately in the patient's case-notes and to consider transfusion in the differential diagnosis.

## Massive or large volume blood transfusions

'Massive transfusion' is the replacement of blood loss equivalent to or greater than the patient's total blood volume in less than 24 hours:

- 70 ml/kg in adults
- 80–90 ml/kg in children or infants.

Morbidity and mortality tend to be high among such patients, not because of the large volumes infused, but because of the initial trauma and the tissue and organ damage secondary to haemorrhage and hypovolaemia.

**It is often the underlying cause and consequences of major haemorrhage that result in complications, rather than the transfusion itself.**

However, administering large volumes of blood and intravenous fluids may itself give rise to the following complications.

## Acidosis

Acidosis in a patient receiving a large volume transfusion is more likely to be the result of inadequate treatment of hypovolaemia than due to the effects of transfusion.

Under normal circumstances, the body can easily neutralize this acid load from transfusion. The routine use of bicarbonate or other alkalizing agents, based on the number of units transfused, is unnecessary.

## Hyperkalaemia

The storage of blood will result in a small increase in extracellular potassium concentration, which will increase the longer it is stored. This rise is rarely of clinical significance, other than in neonatal exchange transfusions.

See pp. 147–151 for neonatal exchange transfusion. Use the freshest blood available in the blood bank and which is less than 7 days old.

## Citrate toxicity and hypocalcaemia

Citrate toxicity is rare, but is most likely to occur during the course of a large volume transfusion of whole blood.

Hypocalcaemia, particularly in combination with hypothermia and acidosis, can cause a reduction in cardiac output, bradycardia, and other dysrhythmias. Citrate is usually rapidly metabolized to bicarbonate.

It is therefore unnecessary to attempt to neutralize the acid load of transfusion. There is very little citrate in red cell concentrates and red cell suspension.

## Depletion of fibrinogen and coagulation factors

Plasma undergoes progressive loss of coagulation factors during storage, particularly Factors V and VIII, unless stored at −25°C or colder.

Red cell concentrates and plasma-reduced units lack coagulation factors which are found in the plasma component.

Dilution of coagulation factors and platelets will occur following administration of large volumes of replacement fluids.

Massive or large volume transfusions can therefore result in disorders of coagulation.

### Management

1 If there is prolongation of the prothrombin time (PT), give ABO-compatible fresh frozen plasma in a dose of 15 ml/kg.

2 If the APTT is also prolonged, Factor VIII/fibrinogen concentrate is recommended in addition to the fresh frozen plasma. If none is available, give 10–15 units of ABO-compatible cryo-precipitate, which contains Factor VIII and fibrinogen.

## Depletion of platelets

Platelet function is rapidly lost during the storage of whole blood and there is virtually no platelet function after 24 hours.

### Management

1 Give platelet concentrates only when:
   - The patient shows clinical signs of microvascular bleeding: i.e. bleeding and oozing from mucous membranes, wounds, raw surfaces and catheter sites
   - The patient's platelet count falls below 50 x $10^9$/L.

2 Give sufficient platelet concentrates to stop the microvascular bleeding and to maintain an adequate platelet count.

3 Consider platelet transfusion in cases where the platelet count falls below 20 x $10^9$/L, even if there is no clinical evidence of bleeding, because there is a danger of hidden bleeding, such as into the brain tissue.

4 The prophylactic use of platelet concentrates in patients receiving large volume blood transfusions is not recommended.

## Disseminated intravascular coagulation

Disseminated intravascular coagulation (DIC) is the abnormal activation of the coagulation and fibrinolytic systems, resulting in the consumption of coagulation factors and platelets.

DIC may develop during the course of a massive blood transfusion, although its cause is less likely to be due to the transfusion itself than related to the underlying reason for transfusion, such as:

- Hypovolaemic shock
- Trauma
- Obstetric complications.

### Management

Treatment should be directed at correcting the underlying cause and at correction of the coagulation problems as they arise. See pp. 115–117 and 130–131.

## Hypothermia

The rapid administration of large volumes of blood or replacement fluids directly from the refrigerator can result in a significant reduction in body temperature. See p. 169.

### Management

If there is evidence of hypothermia, care should be taken during large volume infusions of blood or intravenous fluids.

## Microaggregates

White cells and platelets can aggregate together in stored whole blood, forming microaggregates.

During transfusion, particularly a massive transfusion, these microaggregates embolize to the lung and their presence there has been implicated in the development of adult respiratory distress syndrome (ARDS). However, ARDS following transfusion is most likely to be primarily caused by tissue damage from hypovolaemic shock.

### Management

1   Filters are available to remove microaggregates, but there is little evidence that their use prevents this syndrome.

2   The use of buffy coat-depleted packed red cells will decrease the likelihood of ARDS.

**Notes**

# Clinical decisions on transfusion

## Key points

1 Used correctly, transfusion can be life-saving. Inappropriate use can endanger life.

2 The decision to transfuse blood or blood products should always be based on a careful assessment of clinical and laboratory indications that transfusion is necessary to save life or prevent significant morbidity.

3 Transfusion is only one element in the patient's management.

4 Prescribing decisions should be based on national guidelines on the clinical use of blood, taking individual patient needs into account. However, responsibility for the decision to transfuse ultimately rests with individual clinicians.

# Assessing the need for transfusion

The decision to transfuse blood or blood products should always be based on a careful assessment of clinical and laboratory indications that transfusion is necessary to save life or prevent significant morbidity.

Transfusion is only one element of the patient's management. See below for a summary of the main factors in determining whether transfusion may be required in addition to supportive management and treatment of the underlying condition.

---

**FACTORS DETERMINING THE NEED FOR TRANSFUSION**

**Blood loss**
- External bleeding
- Internal bleeding – non-traumatic: e.g.
  - Peptic ulcer
  - Varices
  - Ectopic pregnancy
  - Antepartum haemorrhage
  - Ruptured uterus
- Internal bleeding – traumatic:
  - Chest
  - Spleen
  - Pelvis
  - Femur
- Red cell destruction: e.g. malaria, sepsis, HIV

**Haemolysis:** e.g.
- Malaria
- Sepsis
- Disseminated intravascular coagulation

**Cardiorespiratory state and tissue oxygenation**
- Pulse rate
- Blood pressure
- Respiratory rate
- Capillary refill

---

- Peripheral pulses
- Temperature of extremities
- Dyspnoea
- Cardiac failure
- Angina
- Conscious level
- Urine output

**Assessment of anaemia**

*Clinical*

- Tongue
- Palms
- Eyes
- Nails

*Laboratory*

- Haemoglobin or haematocrit

**Patient's tolerance of blood loss and/or anaemia**

- Age
- Other clinical conditions: e.g.
  - Pre-eclampsic toxaemia
  - Renal failure
  - Cardiorespiratory disease
  - Chronic lung disease
  - Acute infection
  - Diabetes
  - Treatment with beta-blockers

**Anticipated need for blood**

- Is surgery or anaesthesia anticipated?
- Is bleeding continuing, stopped or likely to recur?
- Is haemolysis continuing?

Prescribing decisions should be based on national guidelines on the clinical use of blood, taking individual patient needs into account. They should also be based on knowledge of local patterns of illness, the resources available for managing patients and the safety and availability of blood and intravenous replacement fluids. However, responsibility for the decision to transfuse ultimately rests with individual clinicians.

## PRESCRIBING BLOOD: A CHECKLIST FOR CLINICIANS

Before prescribing blood or blood products for a patient, ask yourself the following questions.

1   What improvement in the patient's clinical condition am I aiming to achieve?

2   Can I minimize blood loss to reduce this patient's need for transfusion?

3   Are there any other treatments I should give before making the decision to transfuse, such as intravenous replacement fluids and oxygen?

4   What are the specific clinical or laboratory indications for transfusion for this patient?

5   What are the risks of transmitting HIV, hepatitis, syphilis or other infectious agents through the blood products that are available for this patient?

6   Do the benefits of transfusion outweigh the risks for this particular patient?

7   What other options are there if no blood is available in time?

8   Will a trained person monitor this patient and respond immediately if any acute transfusion reactions occur?

9   Have I recorded my decision and reasons for transfusion on the patient's chart and the blood request form?

Finally, if in doubt, ask yourself the following question:

10  If this blood was for myself or my child, would I accept the transfusion in these circumstances?

**Notes**

# General medicine

1   The prevention and treatment of anaemia is one of the most important means of avoiding unnecessary transfusion.

2   Transfusion is rarely needed for chronic anaemia, but chronic anaemia increases the need for transfusion when the patient experiences sudden loss of red cells from bleeding, haemolysis, pregnancy or childbirth.

3   The principles of treatment of anaemia are:
   - Treat the underlying cause of the anaemia
   - Optimize all the components of the oxygen delivery system in order to improve the oxygen supply to the tissues
   - Transfuse only if anaemia is severe enough to reduce the oxygen supply so that it is inadequate for the patient's needs.

4   Treat suspected malaria as a matter of urgency. Starting treatment promptly may save the patient's life.

5   Provided the blood supply is safe, in $\beta$ thalassaemia major, haemoglobin levels should be maintained at 10–12 g/dl by periodic small transfusions. Specific precautions against infections and iron overload should be used.

6   In cases of disseminated intravascular coagulation, rapid treatment or removal of the cause, together with supportive care, is essential. Transfusion may be required until the underlying cause has been dealt with.

# Blood, oxygen and the circulation

In order to ensure a constant supply of oxygen to the tissues and organs of the body, four important steps must take place.

1 Oxygen transfer from the lungs into the blood plasma.

2 Oxygen storage on the haemoglobin molecule in the red cells.

3 Oxygen transport to the tissues of the body via the circulation.

4 Oxygen release from the blood to the tissues, where it can be utilized.

The overall supply of oxygen to the tissues is dependent on:
- Haemoglobin concentration
- Degree of saturation of haemoglobin with oxygen
- Cardiac output.

## The normal haemoglobin range

The normal haemoglobin range is the range of haemoglobin concentrations in healthy individuals. It is:
- An indicator of good health
- A worldwide standard that varies only with age, gender, pregnancy and altitude.

### Criteria for anaemia based on normal haemoglobin range at sea level

| Age/gender | Normal Hb | Anaemic if Hb less than: (g/dl) |
|---|---|---|
| Birth (full-term) | 13.5–18.5 | 13.5 (Hct 34%) |
| Children: 2–6 months | 9.5–13.5 | 9.5 (Hct 28%) |
| Children: 6 months–2 years | | |
| Children: 2–6 years | 11.0–14.0 | 11.0 (Hct 33%) |
| Children: 6–12 years | 11.5–15.5 | 11.5 (Hct 34%) |
| Adult males | 13.0–17.0 | 13.0 (Hct 39%) |
| Adult females: non-pregnant | 12.0–15.0 | 12.0 (Hct 36%) |
| Adult females: pregnant | | |
| First trimester: 0–12 weeks | 11.0–14.0 | 11.0 (Hct 33%) |
| Second trimester: 13–28 weeks | 10.5–14.0 | 10.5 (Hct 31%) |
| Third trimester: 29 weeks–term | 11.0–14.0 | 11.0 (Hct 33%) |

The haemoglobin values shown on p. 85 simply define anaemia. They are often used as thresholds for investigation and treatment, but are **not** indications for transfusion.

The haemoglobin concentration is affected by:

- Amount of circulating haemoglobin
- Blood volume.

## Anaemia

The rate at which anaemia develops usually determines the severity of symptoms.

**Moderate** anaemia may cause no symptoms, especially when due to a chronic process. Nevertheless, it reduces the patient's reserves to adjust to an acute event such as haemorrhage, infection or childbirth.

**Severe** anaemia, whether acute or chronic, is an important factor in reducing the patient's tissue oxygen supply to critical levels. In this situation, urgent treatment is required and the need for transfusion should be assessed.

### Chronic anaemia
### Causes

In chronic blood loss, small amounts of blood are lost from the circulation over a long period of time and normovolaemia is maintained.

### Effects

Chronic blood loss typically results in iron deficiency anaemia which reduces the oxygen-carrying capacity of the blood.

↓ Haemoglobin x ↑ Saturation x ↑ Cardiac output = ↓ Oxygen supply to tissues

### Compensatory responses

- Cardiac output increases
- Oxygen dissociation curve of haemoglobin shifts to increase oxygen release
- Blood viscosity reduces: increased flow
- Fluid retention

## CAUSES OF ANAEMIA

### Increased loss of red blood cells

- Acute blood loss: haemorrhage from trauma, surgery or obstetric haemorrhage
- Chronic blood loss, usually from gastrointestinal, urinary or reproductive tracts: parasitic infestation, malignancy, inflammatory disorders, menorrhagia

### Decreased production of normal red blood cells

- Nutritional deficiencies: iron, $B_{12}$, folate, malnutrition, malabsorption
- Viral infections: HIV
- Bone marrow failure: aplastic anaemia, malignant infiltration of bone marrow, leukaemia
- Reduced erythropoietin production: chronic renal failure
- Chronic illness
- Lead poisoning

### Increased destruction of red blood cells (haemolysis)

- Infections: bacterial, viral, parasitic
- Drugs: e.g. dapsone
- Autoimmune disorders: warm and cold antibody haemolytic disease
- Inherited disorders: sickle cell disease, thalassaemia, G6PD deficiency, spherocytosis
- Haemolytic disease of the newborn (HDN)
- Other disorders: disseminated intravascular coagulation, haemolytic uraemic syndrome, thrombotic thrombocytopenic purpura

### Increased demand for red blood cells

- Pregnancy
- Lactation

### Clinical features

Chronic anaemia may cause few clinical symptoms or signs until a very low haemoglobin concentration is reached. However, the clinical features of anaemia may become apparent at an earlier stage when there is:

- Limited capacity to mount a compensatory response: e.g. significant cardiovascular or respiratory disease
- Increase in demand for oxygen: e.g. infection, pain, fever, exercise
- Further reduction in oxygen supply: e.g. blood loss, pneumonia.

# Acute anaemia

## Causes

Acute blood loss: haemorrhage from:

- Trauma
- Surgery
- Obstetric haemorrhage.

## Effects

- Blood volume falls (hypovolaemia)
- Total haemoglobin in the circulation falls

Leading to:

- Reduced oxygen transport
- Reduced oxygen storage
- Reduced oxygen delivery.

---

$\downarrow$ Haemoglobin x $\downarrow$ Saturation x $\downarrow$ Cardiac output = $\downarrow\downarrow$ Oxygen supply to tissues

---

## Compensatory responses

- Restoration of plasma volume
- Restoration of cardiac output
- Circulatory compensation
- Stimulation of ventilation
- Changes in the oxygen dissociation curve
- Hormonal changes
- Synthesis of plasma proteins.

## Clinical features

The clinical features of haemorrhage are largely determined by:

- Amount and rate of blood loss.
- Patient's compensatory responses.

---

### Major haemorrhage

---

- Thirst
- Tachycardia
- Reduced blood pressure
- Decreased pulse pressure

- Cool, pale, sweaty skin
- Increased respiratory rate
- Reduced urine output
- Restlessness or confusion

---

**Note**: Some patients may suffer substantial blood loss before showing the typical clinical features.

## HISTORY

### Non-specific symptoms of anaemia

- Tiredness/loss of energy
- Light-headedness
- Shortness of breath
- Ankle swelling
- Headache
- Worsening of any pre-existing symptoms: e.g. angina

### History and symptoms relating to the underlying disorder

- Nutritional deficiency
- Pharmaceutical drug history
- Low socio-economic status
- Family history, ethnic origins (haemoglobinopathy)
- History suggesting high risk of exposure to HIV infection
- Fever, nightsweats
- History of malaria episodes; residence in or travel to malaria endemic area
- Obstetric/gynaecological history, menorrhagia or other vaginal bleeding, type of contraception
- Bleeding from urinary tract
- Bleeding gums, epistaxis, purpura (bone marrow failure)
- Gastrointestinal disturbance: melaena, upper GI bleeding, diarrhoea, weight loss, indigestion

## PHYSICAL EXAMINATION

### Signs of anaemia and clinical decompensation

- Pale mucous membranes
- Rapid breathing
- Tachycardia
- Raised jugular venous pressure
- Heart murmurs
- Ankle oedema
- Postural hypotension
- Altered mental state

### Signs of the underlying disorder

- Weight loss/underweight for height/age
- Angular stomatitis, koilonychia (iron deficiency)
- Jaundice (haemolysis)
- Purpura and bruising (bone marrow failure, platelet disorders)
- Enlarged lymph nodes, hepato-splenomegaly (infection, lympho-proliferative disease, HIV/AIDS)
- Lower leg ulcers (sickle cell anaemia)
- Skeletal deformities (thalassaemia)
- Neurological signs (vitamin $B_{12}$ deficiency)

## Clinical assessment

Clinical assessment should determine the type of anaemia, its severity and the probable cause or causes. A patient may have several causes of anaemia, such as nutritional deficiency, HIV, malaria, parasitic infestation.

## Laboratory investigations

A full blood count, examination of the blood film and red cell indices will generally enable the cause of the anaemia to be determined (see p. 92):

- Further investigations may be required to distinguish iron and folate deficiency from other conditions with similar characteristics, such as β thalassaemia
- Screening for G6PD deficiency or abnormal haemoglobin may be needed
- The physical findings, examination of the blood film, a sickle test and haemoglobin electrophoresis will detect most common types of inherited haemoglobinopathies
- The presence of reticulocytes (immature red cells) on the blood film indicates that there is rapid production of red cells
- The absence of reticulocytes in an anaemic patient should prompt a search for bone marrow dysfunction due to infiltration, infection, primary failure or deficiency of haematinics.

## Management

The treatment of anaemia will vary according to the cause, rate of development and degree of compensation to the anaemia. This requires a detailed assessment of the individual patient. However, the principles of treatment of all anaemias are as follows.

1 Treat the underlying cause of the anaemia and monitor the response (see p. 93).

2 If the patient has inadequate oxygenation of the tissues, optimize all the components of the oxygen delivery system to improve the oxygen supply to the tissues.

3 Transfuse only if anaemia is severe enough to reduce the oxygen supply so that it is inadequate for the patient's needs:
- Transfusion in megaloblastic anaemia can be dangerous because poor myocardial function may make the patient likely to develop heart failure
- Restrict transfusion for immune haemolysis to patients with potentially life-threatening anaemia: antibodies in the patient's serum may haemolyse transfused red cells and transfusion may worsen the destruction of the patient's own red cells.

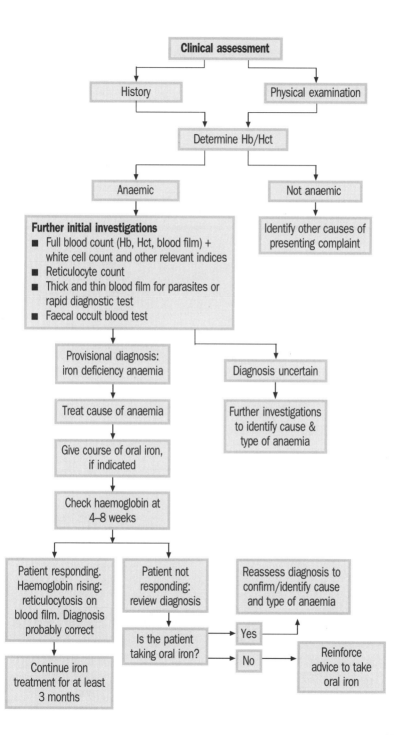

| BLOOD FILM | RED CELL INDICES | CAUSE |
|---|---|---|
| Microcytic, hypochromic with abnormal red cells | ■ Low mean cell volume (MCV)<br>■ Low mean cell haemoglobin (MCH)<br>■ Low mean cell haemoglobin concentration (MCHC) | **Acquired**<br>■ Iron deficiency<br>■ Sideroblastic anaemia<br>■ Anaemia of chronic disorder<br><br>**Congenital**<br>■ Thalassaemia<br>■ Sideroblastic anaemia |
| Macrocytic, normochromic | Increased MCV | **With megaloblastic marrow**<br>■ Deficiency of vitamin $B_{12}$ or folic acid<br><br>**With normoblastic marrow**<br>■ Alcohol excess<br>■ Myelodysplasia |
| Macrocytic polychromasia | Increased MCV | Haemolytic anaemia |
| Normocytic, normochromic | Normal MCV, MCH, MCHC | ■ Chronic disorder<br>— Infection<br>— Malignancy<br>— Autoimmune disorders<br>■ Renal failure<br>■ Hypothyroidism<br>■ Hypopituitarism<br>■ Aplastic anaemia<br>■ Red cell aplasia<br>■ Marrow infiltration |
| Leuco-erythroblastic | Indices may be abnormal due to early and numerous forms of red and white cells | ■ Myelodysplasia<br>■ Leukaemia<br>■ Metastatic cancer<br>■ Myelofibrosis<br>■ Severe infections |

**Note**: MCV is reliable only if calculated using a well-calibrated electronic blood cell counter

## TREATMENT OF CHRONIC ANAEMIA

1  Exclude the possibility of a haemoglobinopathy.

2  Correct any identified cause of blood loss:
   - Treat helminthic or other infections
   - Deal with any local bleeding sources
   - Stop anticoagulant treatment, if possible
   - Stop drugs that are gastric mucosal irritants: e.g. aspirin, non-steroidal anti-inflammatory drugs (NSAIDs)
   - Stop anti-platelet drugs e.g. aspirin, NSAIDs.

3  Give oral iron (ferrous sulphate 200 mg three times per day for an adult; ferrous sulphate 15 mg/kg/day for a child). Continue this treatment for three months or one month after haemoglobin concentration has returned to normal. The haemoglobin level should rise by about 2 g/dl within about 3 weeks. If it does not, review the diagnosis and treatment.

4  Correct identified vitamin deficiencies with oral folic acid (5 mg daily) and vitamin $B_{12}$ (hydroxocobalamin) by injection.

5  Combined tablets of iron and folic acid are useful if there is deficiency of both. Other multi-component preparations for anaemia have no advantages and are often very expensive.

6  Treat malaria with effective antimalarial drugs, taking local resistance patterns into account. Give malaria prophylaxis only where there are specific indications.

7  If evidence of haemolysis, review the drug treatment and, if possible, stop drugs that might be the cause.

8  Check if the patient is on any marrow-suppressing drugs and stop, if possible.

## Severe (decompensated) anaemia

An adult with well-compensated anaemia may have few or no symptoms or signs.

### Causes of decompensation

1  Heart or lung disease that limits the compensatory responses.

2 Increased demand for oxygen:
- Infection
- Pain
- Fever
- Exercise.

3 Acute reduction in oxygen supply:
- Acute blood loss/haemolysis
- Pneumonia.

## Signs of acute decompensation

The severely decompensated patient develops clinical features of inadequate tissue oxygen supply, despite supportive measures and treatment of the underlying cause of the anaemia:

- Mental status changes
- Diminished peripheral pulses
- Congestive cardiac failure
- Hepatomegaly
- Poor peripheral perfusion (capillary refill greater than 2 seconds).

A patient with these clinical signs needs urgent treatment as there is a high risk of death due to insufficient oxygen-carrying capacity.

The clinical signs of hypoxia with severe anaemia may be very similar to those of other causes of respiratory distress, such as an acute infection or an asthmatic attack. These other causes, if present, should be identified and treated, before deciding to transfuse.

---

### TREATMENT OF SEVERE (DECOMPENSATED) ANAEMIA

1 Treat bacterial chest infection aggressively.

2 Give oxygen by mask.

3 Correct fluid balance. If giving intravenous fluids, take care not to put patient into cardiac failure.

4 Decide whether red cell transfusion is (or may be) needed.

5 Use red cells, if available, rather than whole blood to minimize the volume and the oncotic effect of the infusion.

---

Blood transfusion should only be considered when the anaemia is likely to cause, or has already caused, a reduction in the oxygen supply to a level that is inadequate for the patient's needs.

## TRANSFUSION IN SEVERE (DECOMPENSATED) ANAEMIA

1 Do not transfuse more than necessary. If one unit of red cells is enough to correct symptoms, do not give two units. Remember that:
  - The aim is to give the patient sufficient haemoglobin to relieve hypoxia
  - The dose should be matched to the patient's size and blood volume
  - The haemoglobin content of a 450 ml unit of blood may vary from 45 g to 75 g.

2 Patients with severe anaemia may be precipitated into cardiac failure by infusion of blood or other fluids. If transfusion is necessary, give one unit, preferably of red cell concentrate, over 2 to 4 hours and give a rapid acting diuretic (e.g. frusemide, 40 mg IM).

3 Reassess the patient and, if symptoms of severe anaemia persist, give a further 1–2 units.

4 It is not necessary to restore the haemoglobin concentration to normal levels. Raise it enough to relieve the clinical condition.

# Malaria

The diagnosis and treatment of malaria and any associated complications are a matter of urgency as death can occur within 48 hours in non-immune individuals.

Malaria presents as a non-specific acute febrile illness and cannot be reliably distinguished from many other causes of fever on clinical grounds.

The differential diagnosis must therefore consider other infections and causes of fever.

- The clinical manifestations may be modified by partial immunity acquired by previous infection or sub-curative doses of antimalarial drugs
- Since fever is often irregular or intermittent, history of fever over the last 48 hours is important
- Malaria in pregnancy is more severe and is dangerous for mother and fetus; partially immune pregnant women, especially primagravidae, are also susceptible to severe anaemia due to malaria
- Young children who have not yet developed some immunity to the parasite are at particular risk.

## CLINICAL FEATURES OF SEVERE *FALCIPARUM* MALARIA

**May occur alone, or more commonly, in combination in same patient**

- Cerebral malaria, defined as unrousable coma not attributable to any other cause
- Generalized convulsions
- Severe normocytic anaemia
- Hypoglycaemia
- Metabolic acidosis with respiratory distress
- Fluid and electrolyte disturbances
- Acute renal failure
- Acute pulmonary oedema and adult respiratory distress syndrome
- Circulatory collapse, shock, septicaemia ('algid malaria')
- Abnormal bleeding
- Jaundice
- Haemoglobinuria
- High fever
- Hyperparasitaemia

A bad prognosis is indicated by confusion or drowsiness, with extreme weakness (prostration)

## DIAGNOSIS

- High index of suspicion
- Travel history indicative of exposure in endemic area or possible infection through transfusion or injection
- Examination of thin and preferably thick films of peripheral blood by microscopy
- Dipstick antigen test, if available: e.g.
  - ParasightF test (*falciparum* malaria only)
  - ICT test (*falciparum* and *vivax* malaria)
- High parasite density in non-immune people indicates severe disease, but severe malaria can develop even with low parasitaemia; very rarely, blood film may be negative
- Repeat blood count and blood film every 4–6 hours

| MANAGEMENT | TRANSFUSION |
|---|---|
| 1  Promptly treat infection and any associated complications, following local treatment regimes. | **Adults, including pregnant women** Consider transfusion if haemoglobin <7 g/dl (see p. 126 for transfusion in chronic anaemia in pregnancy) |
| 2  Where index of suspicion, treat urgently on basis of clinical assessment alone, if delays in laboratory investigations are likely. | **Children** ■ Transfuse if haemoglobin <4 g/dl ■ Transfuse if haemoglobin 4–6 g/dl and clinical features of: — Hypoxia — Acidosis — Impaired consciousness — Hyperparasitaemia (>20%) |
| 3  Correct dehydration and hypoglycaemia: avoid precipitating pulmonary oedema with fluid overload. | |
| 4  Specific treatments for serious complications: ■ Transfusion to correct life-threatening anaemia ■ Haemofiltration or dialysis for renal failure ■ Anticonvulsants for fits. | |

**In endemic malarial areas, there is a high risk of transmitting malaria by transfusion. Give the transfused patient routine treatment for malaria.**

# HIV/AIDS

HIV infection is associated with anaemia due to a variety of causes. Around 80% of AIDS patients will have a haemoglobin level less than 10 g/dl. The management of anaemia in HIV infection is based on treating associated conditions.

## Transfusion

When anaemia is severe, the decision to transfuse should be made using the same criteria as for any other patient.

# Glucose-6-phosphate dehydrogenase (G6PD) deficiency

G6PD deficiency is commonly asymptomatic and can cause jaundice and anaemia precipitated by infection, drugs or chemicals.

Haemolysis will stop once the cells that are most deficient in G6PD have been destroyed. It is important to remove or treat any identified cause.

### Transfusion

1  Transfusion is not required in most cases of G6PD deficiency.

2  Transfusion may be life-saving in severe haemolysis when the haemoglobin continues to fall rapidly.

3  Exchange transfusions are indicated for neonates at risk of kernicterus and who are unresponsive to phototherapy (see pp. 147–153).

# Bone marrow failure

Bone marrow failure is present when the bone marrow is unable to produce adequate cells to maintain normal counts in the peripheral blood. It usually manifests as pancytopenia – reduced levels of two or three of the cellular elements of blood (red cells, white cells, platelets).

Anaemia due to the underlying disease and to treatment may become symptomatic and require red cell replacement.

### MANAGEMENT OF BONE MARROW FAILURE OR SUPPRESSION

1  Treat infection.

2  Maintain fluid balance.

3  Give supportive treatment: e.g. nutrition, pain control.

4  Stop potentially toxic drug treatments.

5  Ensure good nutrition.

6  Treat the underlying condition:
   - Chemotherapy for leukaemia or lymphoma **plus**
   - Irradiation therapy for some conditions
   - Bone marrow transplant for some conditions.

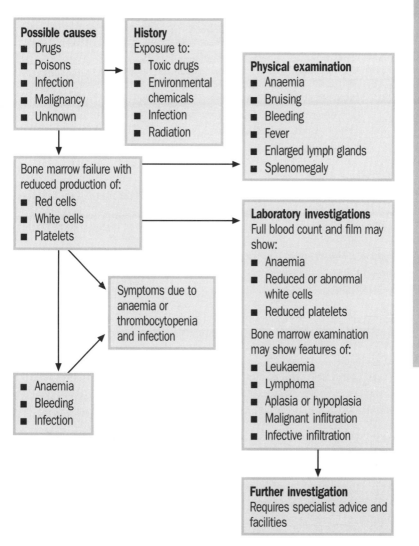

**Possible causes**
- Drugs
- Poisons
- Infection
- Malignancy
- Unknown

**History**
Exposure to:
- Toxic drugs
- Environmental chemicals
- Infection
- Radiation

**Physical examination**
- Anaemia
- Bruising
- Bleeding
- Fever
- Enlarged lymph glands
- Splenomegaly

Bone marrow failure with reduced production of:
- Red cells
- White cells
- Platelets

**Laboratory investigations**
Full blood count and film may show:
- Anaemia
- Reduced or abnormal white cells
- Reduced platelets

Bone marrow examination may show features of:
- Leukaemia
- Lymphoma
- Aplasia or hypoplasia
- Malignant infiltration
- Infective infiltration

Symptoms due to anaemia or thrombocytopenia and infection

- Anaemia
- Bleeding
- Infection

**Further investigation**
Requires specialist advice and facilities

## Transfusion of patients with bone marrow failure or suppression due to chemotherapy

Chemotherapy, irradiation therapy and bone marrow transplant commonly suppress bone marrow further and increase the need for transfusion support with red cells and platelets until remission occurs.

1   If repeated transfusions are likely to be needed, use leucocyte-reduced red cells and platelets, wherever possible, to reduce the risk of reactions and of alloimmunization.

2 Avoid transfusing blood components from any blood relative to prevent the risk of graft-versus-host disease (GvHD) in immunosuppressed patients (see p. 73).

3 Some immunosuppressed patients are at risk of cytomegalovirus (CMV) infection transmitted by blood transfusion. This can be avoided or reduced by transfusing blood that is tested and contains no CMV antibodies or by using leucocyte-depleted blood components.

### Red cell transfusion

Anaemia due to the underlying disease and to treatment may become symptomatic and require red cell replacement. A red cell component is preferable to whole blood as the patient is at risk of circulatory overload.

### Platelet transfusion

Platelet transfusion may be given either to control or prevent bleeding due to thrombocytopenia.

The adult 'dose' of platelets should contain at least $240 \times 10^9$ platelets. This can be provided by infusing the platelets separated from 4–6 units of whole blood or obtained from one donor by plateletpheresis.

### Platelet transfusion to control bleeding

1 Set a platelet transfusion regime for each patient. The aim is to balance the risk of haemorrhage against the risks of repeated platelet transfusion (infection and alloimmunization).

2 Clinical signs such as mucosal or retinal haemorrhage, or purpura in a patient with a low platelet count, generally indicate the need for platelet transfusion to control bleeding. They should also prompt a check for the causes, such as infection.

3 Often one platelet transfusion will control bleeding, but repeated transfusions over several days may be needed.

4 Failure to control bleeding may be due to:
   ■ Infection
   ■ Splenomegaly
   ■ Antibodies against leucocytes or platelet antigens
   ■ Failure to control the primary condition.

5 Increasing the frequency of platelet transfusion and occasionally the use of HLA-compatible platelet concentrates may help to control bleeding.

### Platelet transfusion to prevent bleeding

1 Platelets are usually not given for stable afebrile patients, provided the count is above 10 x 10$^9$/L.

2 If the patient has a fever and possible infection, many clinicians adopt a higher threshold of 20 x 10$^9$/L.

3 If the patient is stable, platelet transfusions should be given to maintain the platelet count at the chosen level; transfusion every 2 or 3 days is often sufficient.

## Sickle cell disease

### Acute crises

Acute crises include:

- Vaso-occlusive crises, leading to pain and infarction
- Splenic sequestration crises
- Aplastic crises due to infections: e.g. parvovirus, folate deficiency
- Haemolytic crises (occur rarely).

### Chronic complications

Chronic complications are the result of prolonged or repeated ischaemia leading to infarction. They include:

- Skeletal abnormalities and delayed puberty
- Neurological loss due to stroke
- Hyposplenism
- Chronic renal failure
- Impotence following priapism
- Loss of lung function
- Visual loss.

### Laboratory investigations

Laboratory investigations to detect anaemia, characteristic abnormalities of the red blood cells and the presence of abnormal haemoglobin:

- Haemoglobin concentration: Hb of 5–11 g/dl (usually low in relation to symptoms of anaemia)
- Blood film to detect sickle cells, target cells and reticulocytosis
- Sickle solubility or slide test to identify sickle cells
- HbF quantitation to detect elevation of HbF
- Haemoglobin electrophoresis to identify abnormal haemoglobin patterns. In homozygous HbSS, no normal HbA is detectable.

## Management

The main aims are:

- To prevent crises
- To minimize long-term damage when a crisis does occur.

### PREVENTION OF SICKLE CRISIS

1. Avoid precipitating factors:
   - Dehydration
   - Hypoxia
   - Infection
   - Cold
   - Slowed circulation.

2. Give folic acid 5 mg daily orally **long-term.**

3. Give penicillin:
   - 2.4 million iu benzathine penicillin IM **long-term**
   
   *or*
   - Penicillin V 250 mg daily orally **long-term.**

4. Vaccinate against *pneumococcus* and, if possible, hepatitis B.

5. Recognize and treat malaria promptly. Haemolysis due to malaria may precipitate a sickle crisis.

6. Treat other infections promptly.

7. Consider whether regular transfusion is indicated.

### TREATMENT OF SICKLE CRISIS

1. Rehydrate with oral fluids and, if necessary intravenous normal saline.

2. Treat systemic acidosis with IV bicarbonate, if necessary.

3. Correct hypoxia: give supplemental oxygen, if required.

4. Give effective pain relief: strong analgesics, including opiates (i.e. morphine), are likely to be needed.

5. Treat malaria, if infected.

6. Treat bacterial infection with the best available antibiotic in full dose.

7. Give transfusion, if required.

## Transfusion and exchange transfusion in the prevention and treatment of sickle crisis

### Prevention of crises and long-term disability

1  Regular red cell transfusion has a role in reducing the frequency of crises in (homozygous) SCD and preventing recurrent strokes. It may also assist in preventing recurrent life-threatening acute lung syndrome and chronic sickle cell lung disease.

2  Transfusion is not indicated purely to raise a low haemoglobin level. Patients with SCD are well-adapted to haemoglobin levels of 7–10 g/dl and are at risk of hyperviscosity if the haemoglobin is raised significantly above the patient's normal baseline without a reduction in the proportion of sickle cells.

3  Aim to maintain a sufficient proportion of normal HbA (about 30% or more) in the circulation to suppress the production of HbS-containing red cells and minimize the risk of sickling episodes.

4  Stroke occurs in 7–8% of children with SCD and is a major cause of morbidity. Regular transfusions can reduce recurrence rates for stroke from 46–90% down to less than 10%.

5  Regularly-transfused patients are at risk of iron overload (see p. 107), transfusion-transmissible infections and alloimmunization.

### Treatment of crises and severe anaemia

1  Transfusion is indicated in severe acute anaemia (haemoglobin concentration of <5 g/dl or >2 g/dl below the patient's normal baseline).

2  Prompt transfusion in sequestration crisis and aplastic crisis can be life-saving. Aim for a haemoglobin level of 7–8 g/dl only.

#### Sequestration crisis

1  The patient presents with the equivalent of hypovolaemic shock due to loss of blood from the circulation into the spleen.

2  The circulating blood volume must be urgently restored with intravenous fluid.

3  Blood transfusion is usually needed.

#### Aplastic crisis

Aplastic crisis is usually triggered by infection: e.g. parvovirus. There is transient acute bone marrow failure and transfusions may be needed until the marrow recovers.

## Management of pregnancy and anaesthesia in patients with sickle cell disease

1  Routine transfusions during pregnancy may be considered for patients with a bad obstetric history or frequent crises.

2  Preparation for delivery or surgery with anaesthesia may include transfusion to bring the proportion of HbS below 30%.

3  Anaesthetic techniques and supportive care should ensure that blood loss, hypoxia, dehydration and acidosis are minimized.

### Sickle cell trait

1  Patients with sickle cell trait (HbAS) are asymptomatic, may have a normal haemoglobin level and the red cells may appear normal on a blood film.

2  Crises may be provoked by dehydration and hypoxia.

3  Anaesthesia, pregnancy or delivery should be managed with care in known carriers.

# Thalassaemias

| Condition | Genetic defect | Clinical features |
|---|---|---|
| Homozygous β thalassaemia (β thalassaemia major) | β chain suppression or deletion | Severe anaemia: Hb <7 g/dl Dependent on transfusion |
| Heterozygous β thalassaemia (β thalassaemia minor trait) | β chain deletion | Asymptomatic: mild anaemia: Hb >10 g/dl |
| Thalassaemia intermedia | β chain suppression or deletion | Heterogeneous: ranges from asymptomatic to resembling β thalassaemia major: Hb 7–10 g/dl |
| Homozygous α thalassaemia | All 4 α globin chains deleted | Fetus does not survive (hydrops fetalis) |
| α thalassaemia minor | Loss of two or three α genes | Usually mild or moderate |
| α thalassaemia trait | Loss of one or two α genes | Symptomless: mild microcytic, hypochromic anaemia |

The differentiation at presentation between thalassaemia intermedia and major is essential in determining appropriate treatment. A careful analysis of the clinical, haematological, genetic and molecular data (see below), may assist in the differential diagnosis.

| | Major | Intermedia | Minor |
|---|---|---|---|
| Haemoglobin (g/dl) | <7 | 7–10 | >10 |
| Reticulocytes (%) | 2–15 | 2–10 | <5 |
| Nucleated red cells | ++/++++ | +/+++ | 0 |
| Red cell morphology | ++++ | ++ | + |
| Jaundice | +++ | +/++ | 0 |
| Splenomegaly | ++++ | ++/+++ | 0 |
| Skeletal changes | ++/+++ | +/++ | 0 |

## Clinical features
### Thalassaemia major
1 β thalassaemia major presents within the first year of life, with failure to thrive and anaemia. Without effective treatment, it usually leads to death before the age of ten years.

2 Patients are reliant on transfusion to maintain a haemoglobin level sufficient to oxygenate the tissues.

3 Iron accumulates in the body due to the destruction of red cells, increased absorption and red cell transfusion. This leads to cardiac failure, hormone deficiencies, cirrhosis and eventually death, unless iron chelation therapy is instigated (see p. 108).

## Laboratory findings
### Thalassaemia major
1 Severe microcytic, hypochromic anaemia.

2 Blood film: red cells are microcytic and hypochromic with target cells, basophilic stippling and nucleated red cells.

3 Haemoglobin electrophoresis: absent HbA with raised HbF and $HbA_2$.

### Thalassaemia intermedia, minor or trait
1 Microcytic, hypochromic anaemia: normal iron, TIBC.

2 Haemoglobin electrophoresis: depends on variant.

## MANAGEMENT OF THALASSAEMIA MAJOR

1   Transfusion.

2   Chelation therapy.

3   Vitamin C: 200 mg by mouth to promote iron excretion, on the day of iron chelation only.

4   Folic acid: 5 mg day by mouth.

5   Splenectomy may be required to reduce the transfusion requirement. It should not be performed in children under 6 years of age because of high risk of infections.

6   Long-term penicillin.

7   Vaccinate against:
    - Hepatitis B
    - *Pneumococcus.*

8   Endocrine replacement for diabetes, pituitary failure.

9   Vitamin D and calcium for parathyroid failure.

## TRANSFUSION IN THALASSAEMIA MAJOR

1   Planned blood transfusions can save life and improve its quality by helping to avoid the complications of hypertrophied marrow and early cardiac failure.

2   Give only essential transfusions to minimize iron overload, which eventually leads to iron accumulation, damaging the heart, endocrine system and liver.

3   Aim to transfuse red cells in sufficient quantity and frequently enough to suppress erythropoiesis.

4   Where the risks of transfusion are judged to be small and iron chelation is available, target haemoglobin levels of 10.0–12.0 g/dl may be applied. It is not advisable to exceed a haemoglobin level of 15 g/dl.

5   Small transfusions are preferred because they need less blood and suppress red cell production more effectively.

6   Splenectomy may be required and will usually reduce the transfusion requirement.

## PROBLEMS ASSOCIATED WITH REPEATED RED CELL TRANSFUSIONS

| | |
|---|---|
| Alloimmunization | If possible, give red cells matched for red cell phenotypes, especially Kell, RhD and RhE, that readily stimulate clinically significant antibodies in the recipient |
| Febrile non-haemolytic transfusion reactions | ■ Consistent use of leucocyte-depleted red cell transfusions can delay onset or severity<br>■ Reduce symptoms by premedication with paracetamol:<br>— Adults: 1 g orally one hour before transfusion. Repeat, if necessary, after starting transfusion<br>— Children over 1 month: 30–40 mg/kg/24 hours in 4 doses |
| Hyperviscosity | Can precipitate vascular occlusion:<br>■ Maintain the circulating fluid volume<br>■ Transfuse only to maximum haemoglobin level of 12 g/dl<br>■ Exchange red cell transfusion may be required to achieve a sufficient reduction of HbS red cells without increasing viscosity |
| Infection | If blood has not been tested for hepatitis:<br>■ Administer hepatitis B vaccine to non-immune patients<br>■ Administer HAV vaccine to all anti-HCV positive thalassaemics |
| Iron overload | ■ Give only essential transfusions<br>■ Give desferrioxamine (see p. 108) |
| Splenectomy | ■ Do not perform in children younger than 6 years<br>■ Vaccinate against *pneumococcus* 2–4 weeks prior to splenectomy<br>■ Yearly administration of influenza vaccine is recommended in splenectomized patients<br>■ The efficacy and utility of vaccination against *N. meningitidis* is not as clear as for *S. pneumonia*<br>■ Lifelong penicillin prophylaxis is needed |
| Venous access | See p. 184 on preserving venous access |

## IRON CHELATION FOR TRANSFUSION-DEPENDENT PATIENTS

1 Give subcutaneous infusion of desferrioxamine: 25–50 mg/kg/day over 8–12 hours, 5–7 days per week. Dose adjustment should be conducted on an individual basis.

Young children should be started on a dose of 25–35 mg/kg/day, increasing to a maximum of 40 mg/kg/day after 5 years of age and increasing further up to 50 mg/kg/day after growth has ceased.

2 Give vitamin C up to 200 mg/day orally one hour after initiating chelation.

3 Undertake splenectomy, if indicated (but not before 6 years of age).

**In exceptional cases, under careful monitoring**
Give desferrioxamine 60 mg/kg by intravenous infusion over 24 hours, using the patient's subcutaneous infusion pump with the butterfly inserted into the drip tubing. **Do not put desferrioxamine into the blood pack.**

*Or*

Give desferrioxamine 50–70 mg/kg/day in a continuous intravenous infusion via an implanted catheter device. This method should be used only for patients with very high iron levels and/or other iron-related complications.

Close monitoring for ocular and auditory toxicity is strongly recommended. Some patients are unable to take desferrioxamine for medical reasons.

# Bleeding disorders and transfusion

Patients who have an abnormality of platelets or the coagulation/ fibrinolytic system may suffer from severe bleeding due to childbirth, surgery or trauma.

Recognition that a patient may have a bleeding disorder and the correct diagnosis and treatment can influence the timing and type of elective surgery, reduce the need for transfusion and avoid risks to the patient due to bleeding.

A bleeding tendency may be due to:
- Congenital (inherited) disorder of blood vessels, platelets or coagulation factors
- Use of pharmaceutical drugs

- Trauma
- Haemorrhage
- Obstetric complications
- Nutritional deficiencies
- Immunological disorders.

## Clinical assessment

See p. 110. The clinical history is perhaps the most important single component of the investigation of haemostatic function. Where the family history suggests an inherited disorder, construct a family tree, if possible.

## Laboratory investigations

Laboratory investigations should be performed when a bleeding problem is suspected. This is especially important if surgery is planned.

The investigation of the bleeding problem should be as methodical as possible. See p. 111 for a flow chart for the interpretation of routine tests in bleeding disorders.

# Congenital bleeding and clotting disorders

## Deficiencies of Factor VIII and IX
### Clinical features

The clinical characteristics of deficiencies of Factors VIII and IX are identical. Both are X-linked recessive disorders affecting males almost exclusively. The clinical severity of the disorder is determined by the amount of active coagulation factor available.

- In severe cases, there is spontaneous delayed deep soft tissue bleeding, particularly into joints and muscles. Chronic synovitis eventually supervenes, leading to pain, bony deformities and contractures. Bleeding after circumcision is a frequent mode of presentation in babies.
- Moderate or mild haemophilia may cause severe bleeding when tissues are damaged by surgery or trauma.

### Laboratory findings
- Prolongation of activated partial thromboplastin time (APTT)
- Normal prothrombin time.

The abnormal APTT corrects with the addition of normal plasma.

## HISTORY

### Symptoms suggestive of bleeding disorder

- Easy bruising
- Development of purpura
- Nosebleeds
- Excessive bleeding after circumcision, dental extraction or other surgery
- Menorrhagia, frequently accompanied by the passage of clots
- Perinatal haemorrhage
- Dark or bloody stools
- Red urine
- Swollen, painful joints or muscles
- Excessive bleeding after minor scratches
- Bleeding that recurs hours or days after original trauma
- Poor wound healing

### Other symptoms

- Weight loss
- Anorexia
- Fever and night sweats

### Exposure to drugs or chemicals

- Alcohol ingestion
- All current or past drugs used by the patient
- Any exposure to drugs or chemicals at work or in the home

### Family history

- Relatives with a similar condition
- Relatives with any history suggesting bleeding disorder

## PHYSICAL EXAMINATION

### Signs of bleeding or blood loss

- Pale mucous membranes
- Petechial haemorrhages
- Purpura or ecchymoses (bruising)
- Bleeding from mucous membranes
- Muscle haematomas
- Haemarthroses or deformed joints
- Positive faecal occult blood test
- Blood observed at rectal examination

### Other signs

- Splenomegaly
- Hepatomegaly
- Jaundice
- Fever
- Tenderness
- Lymphadenopathy

## INTERPRETATION

Source of bleeding usually suggests the most likely cause:

- Bleeding from mucous membranes suggests low platelet count or platelet abnormalities, von Willebrand's disease or vascular defects
- Muscle and joint bleeding or bruising suggest haemophilia A or B

**Note:** Skin manifestations of bleeding disorders (i.e. petechial haemorrhages or ecchymoses) may be difficult to see in dark-skinned patients. Examination of the mucous membranes, including conjunctivae, oral mucosa and optic fundi, for evidence of bleeding is therefore very important.

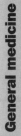

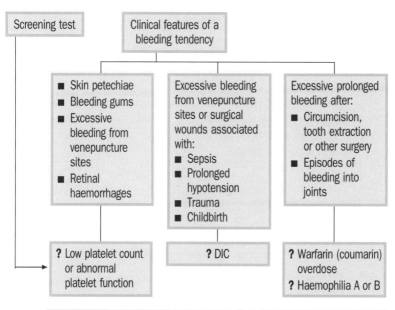

Screening test

Clinical features of a bleeding tendency

- Skin petechiae
- Bleeding gums
- Excessive bleeding from venepuncture sites
- Retinal haemorrhages

Excessive bleeding from venepuncture sites or surgical wounds associated with:
- Sepsis
- Prolonged hypotension
- Trauma
- Childbirth

Excessive prolonged bleeding after:
- Circumcision, tooth extraction or other surgery
- Episodes of bleeding into joints

? Low platelet count or abnormal platelet function

? DIC

? Warfarin (coumarin) overdose
? Haemophilia A or B

| | Thrombocytopenia | Heparin | DIC | Fibrinolytic therapy | von Willebrand's disease | Liver disease | Warfarin | Haemophilia A | Haemophilia B | Massive transfusion |
|---|---|---|---|---|---|---|---|---|---|---|
| **Laboratory investigations: typical results** | | | | | | | | | | |
| Platelet count | ↓ | N | ↓ | N | N/↓ | N/↓ | N | N | N | ↓ |
| Prothrombin time | N | N | ↑ | ↑ | N | ↑ | ↑ | N | N | ↑ |
| Activated partial thromboplastin time | N | ↑ | ↑ | ↑ | N/↑ | ↑ | ↑ | ↑ | ↑ | ↑ |
| Thrombin time | N | ↑ | ↑ | ↑ | N | ↑ | N | N | N | N/↑ |
| Fibrinogen concentration | N | N | ↓ | ↓ | N | ↓ | N | N | N | N/↓ |
| Fibrin degradation products | N | N | ↑ | ↑ | N | N/↑ | N | N | N | N/↑ |

Reversal of prolonged thrombin time by protamine indicates heparin is present

N = Normal

## Management of an acute bleed

1  Avoid anti-platelet agents such as aspirin and non-steroidal anti-inflammatory drugs.

2  Do not give intramuscular injections.

3  Administer coagulation factor concentrates to treat bleeding episodes as quickly as possible. Haemarthroses need strong analgesia, ice packs and immobilization initially. **Never incise joint for haemarthrosis**.

4  Do not incise swellings in haemophiliacs.

5  Start physiotherapy early to minimize loss of joint function.

### *Desmopressin (DDAVP)*

■  May be useful in mild or moderate haemophilia A

■  Not indicated in Factor IX deficiency.

### *Replacement with factor concentrates*

■  Use virus-inactivated factor concentrates to prevent the risk of transmission of HIV and hepatitis B and C

■  If coagulation factor concentrates are not available, use:
— Haemophilia A: Cryoprecipitate
— Haemophilia B: Fresh frozen plasma or liquid plasma.

# von Willebrand's disease

## Clinical features

Deficiency of von Willebrand factor (vWF) is inherited as an autosomal dominant condition. It affects both males and females.

The major clinical manifestation is mucocutaneous bleeding, such as:

■  Epistaxis
■  Easy bruising
■  Menorrhagia
■  Bleeding after dental extractions
■  Post-traumatic bleeding.

## Laboratory investigations

The abnormality of platelet function is best detected by demonstrating a prolonged bleeding time (by the template method) and a prolonged APTT.

## DOSAGE OF FACTOR VIII AND ALTERNATIVES FOR TREATMENT OF HAEMOPHILIA A

| Severity of bleed | Dosage | Supplied as: Factor VIII concentrate (500 iu/bottle) | or Cryoprecipitate* (80–100 iu/pack) |
|---|---|---|---|
| Mild bleed: nose, gums, etc. | 14 iu/kg | 1–2 bottles (adult) | 1 pack/6 kg |
| Moderate bleed: joint, muscle, gastrointestinal tract, surgery | 20 iu/kg | 2–4 bottles (adult) | 1 pack/4 kg |
| Major bleed: e.g. cerebral | 40 iu/kg | 4–6 bottles (adult) | 1 pack/2 kg |
| Prophylaxis for major surgery | 60 iu/kg | 6–10 bottles (adult) | 1 pack/1 kg |

**Note**

\* Cryoprecipitate containing 80–100 iu of Factor VIII, usually obtained from 250 ml of fresh frozen plasma.

1 For a mild, moderate or severe bleed, repeat dose 12-hourly if bleeding persists or swelling is increasing. With more severe bleeds, it is usually necessary to continue treatment with half of total daily dose 12-hourly for 2–3 days or occasionally longer.

2 For prophylaxis for major surgery, start therapy 8 hours before surgery. Continue 12-hourly therapy for 48 hours postoperatively. If no bleeding occurs, scale down gradually over next 3–5 days.

3 As adjunct to factor replacement in mucosal or gastrointestinal bleeding and surgery, give fibrinolytic inhibitor:

Tranexamic acid (oral): 500–1000 mg 3 times/day. Do **not** use for haematuria.

4 In an emergency, use fresh frozen plasma to treat bleeding in haemophiliacs (give 3 packs initially) if none of the above are available.

5 Careful assessment of the patient's fluid intake is important to avoid fluid overload when using fresh frozen plasma or large doses of cryoprecipitate.

## DOSAGE OF FACTOR IX FOR TREATMENT OF HAEMOPHILIA B

| Severity of bleed | Dosage | Supplied as: Factor IX concentrate or (500 iu/bottle) | Fresh frozen plasma |
|---|---|---|---|
| Mild bleed | 15 iu/kg | 2 bottles (adult) | 1 pack/15 kg |
| Major bleed | 20–30 iu/kg | 3–6 bottles (adult) | 1 pack/7.5 kg |

**Note**

1  Repeat in 24 hours if bleeding continues.

2  Factor VIII concentrate and cryoprecipitate are not useful for haemophilia B, so accurate diagnosis is essential.

3  As adjunct to replacement therapy:

  Tranexamic acid (oral): 500–1000 mg 3 times/day, as for haemophilia A.

## Management of von Willebrand's disease

Aim to normalize bleeding time by:

■ Increasing endogenous vWF levels with desmopressin **or**

■ Replacing vWF using intermediate-purity Factor VIII product that is known to contain some vWF or with cryoprecipitate, which also contains vWF.

### Dose regime

Treat as for mild or moderate bleed of haemophilia A, except that the haemostatic dose may be repeated not 12-hourly, but after 24–48 hours, as von Willebrand factor has a longer half-life than Factor VIII.

1  **Desmopressin (DDAVP)**
  0.3–0.4 $\mu$g/kg IV lasts 4–8 hours and avoids the need to use plasma products. The dose can be repeated every 24 hours, but the effect is reduced after some days of treatment.

2  **Factor VIII products**
  Reserve for patients unresponsive to desmopressin. It is essential to use a virally-inactivated product that contains vWF.

3  **Cryoprecipitate**
  Cryoprecipitate is effective, but is not available in virally-inactivated form in most countries.

# Acquired bleeding and clotting disorders

## Disseminated intravascular coagulation

In disseminated intravascular coagulation (DIC), the coagulation and fibrinolytic systems are both activated, leading to deficiencies of the coagulation factors, fibrinogen and platelets.

### Causes

Common causes of DIC include:

- Infection
- Malignancy
- Trauma
- Acute leukaemia
- Eclampsia
- Abruptio placenta
- Amniotic fluid embolism
- Retained products of conception
- Retained dead fetus.

### Clinical features

In severe DIC, there is excessive, uncontrolled bleeding. The lack of platelets and coagulation factors causes:

- Haemorrhage
- Bruising
- Oozing from venepuncture sites.

Microvascular thrombi may cause multiple organ dysfunction leading to:

- Respiratory distress
- Coma
- Renal failure
- Jaundice.

The clinical picture ranges from major haemorrhage, with or without thrombotic complications, to a clinically stable state that can be detected only by laboratory testing.

### Laboratory findings

DIC is characterized by:

- Reduced coagulation factors (so all coagulation tests are prolonged)

- Reduced platelet count (thrombocytopenia)
- Prolonged activated partial thromboplastin time (APTT)
- Prolonged prothrombin time (PT)
- Prolonged thrombin time: particularly helpful in establishing presence or absence of DIC
- Decreased fibrinogen concentration
- Breakdown of products of fibrinogen: fibrin degradation products (FDPs)
- Fragmented red cells on the blood film.

In less acute forms of DIC, sufficient platelets and coagulation factors may be produced to maintain haemostasis, but laboratory tests reveal evidence of fibrinolysis (FDPs).

If laboratory tests are not available, use the following simple clotting test for DIC.

1 Take 2–3 ml of venous blood into a clean plain **glass** test tube (10 x 75 mm).

2 Hold the tube in your closed fist to keep it warm (i.e. body temperature).

3 After 4 minutes, tip the tube slowly to see if a clot is forming. Then tip it again every minute until the blood clots and the tube can be turned upside down.

4 The clot will normally form between 4 and 11 minutes but, in DIC, the blood will remain fluid well beyond 15 to 20 minutes.

### Management
Rapid treatment or removal of the underlying condition is imperative.

> If DIC is suspected, do not delay treatment while waiting for the results of coagulation tests. Treat the cause and use blood products to help control haemorrhage.

### Transfusion
Transfusion support should be given to help control bleeding until the underlying cause has been dealt with and to maintain an adequate platelet count and coagulation factor levels.

## MANAGEMENT OF DISSEMINATED INTRAVASCULAR COAGULATION

1  Monitor:
   - Activated partial thromboplastin time
   - Prothrombin time
   - Thrombin time
   - Platelet count
   - Fibrinogen.

2  Identify and treat or remove the cause of DIC.

3  Give supportive care:
   - Fluids
   - Vasopressor agents
   - Renal, cardiac or ventilatory assistance.

## TRANSFUSION IN DISSEMINATED INTRAVASCULAR COAGULATION

1  If the PT or APTT is prolonged and the patient is bleeding:
   - Replace red cell losses with the freshest whole blood available as it contains fibrinogen and most other coagulation factors

   *and*

   - Give fresh frozen plasma as this contains labile coagulation factors: 1 pack/15 kg body weight (4–5 packs in adults)
   - Repeat FFP according to the clinical response.

2  If fibrinogen is low or the APTT or thrombin time is prolonged, also give cryoprecipitate (to supply fibrinogen and Factor VIII): 1 pack/6 kg (8–10 packs in adults).

3  If the platelet count is less than $50 \times 10^9/L$ and the patient is bleeding, also give platelet concentrates: 4–6 packs (adult).

4  The use of heparin is not recommended in bleeding patients with DIC.

**Note**
Doses are based on the preparation of fresh frozen plasma, cryoprecipitate and platelet concentrates from 450 ml donations.

# Disorders of vitamin K-dependent coagulation factors

Vitamin K is a cofactor for the synthesis of Factors II, VII, IX and X, which takes place in the liver.

Deficiency of vitamin K-dependent coagulation factors may be present in the following conditions:

- Haemorrhagic disease of the newborn (see p. 145)
- Ingestion of coumarin anticoagulants (warfarin)
  Note: when a patient is taking coumarin, starting other drugs (such as some antibiotics) may cause bleeding by displacing warfarin bound to plasma proteins
- Vitamin K deficiency due to inadequate diet or malabsorption
- Liver disease, leading to underproduction of Factors II, VII, IX: a prolonged prothrombin time is usually a feature of severe liver disease with severe loss of hepatocytes.

### Clinical features

Clinically, these disorders usually present with bleeding from the gastrointestinal or urogenital tracts.

### Laboratory findings

- The prothrombin time is prolonged, often severely so
- For patients with liver disease, thrombocytopenia and abnormalities of fibrinogen and fibrinolysis often complicate diagnosis and treatment.

### Management

1 Remove the underlying cause of vitamin K deficiency:
   - Stop anticoagulants (warfarin)
   - Treat malabsorption or dietary deficiency.

2 Replace coagulation factors with fresh frozen plasma, as necessary.

3 Reverse warfarin with intravenous vitamin K if the patient is bleeding and the INR is >4.5. Doses of vitamin K exceeding 1 mg may make the patient refractory to further warfarin for up to 2 weeks. If anticoagulation is still needed, consider doses of 0.1–0.5 mg.

## Bleeding problems associated with surgery

See pp. 160–162.

## Gastrointestinal bleeding

Gastrointestinal bleeding is common and has a significant mortality risk.

## Clinical features

1 Upper gastrointestinal bleeding can present as anaemia due to chronic bleeding, haematemesis (vomiting blood) or melaena (black, altered blood passed from the rectum).

2 Lower gastrointestinal bleeding presents as anaemia with a positive faecal occult blood test or fresh blood in or on the faeces.

3 Peptic ulcer (gastric, duodenal).

4 Oesophageal varices.

5 Gastric carcinoma.

Patients with oesophageal varices, usually due to chronic liver disease, may also have peptic ulcers or erosions.

## Management

1 Resuscitate the patient (see p. 120).

2 Find the source of bleeding (by endoscopy, if possible).

3 Give $H_2$ receptor blockers (e.g. Tagamet, Cimetidine).

4 Stop continued or repeat bleeding by endoscopy or surgical means.

Most patients stop bleeding without surgical or endoscopic intervention. Re-bleeding has a high mortality and is more likely in patients who:

■ Are old
■ Are shocked on admission to hospital
■ Have acute bleeding visible on endoscopy
■ Have gastric (rather than duodenal) ulcer
■ Have liver disease.

## RESUSCITATION AND TRANSFUSION IN ACUTE GASTROINTESTINAL BLEEDING

| Severity of bleed | Clinical features | IV infusion/ transfusion | End point |
|---|---|---|---|
| Mild bleed | Pulse and haemoglobin normal | ■ Maintain intra-venous access until diagnosis is clear<br>■ Ensure blood is available | |
| Moderate bleed | Resting pulse: >100/min **and/or** Haemoglobin <10 g/dl | ■ Replace fluid<br>■ Order 4 units of red cells | Maintain Hb >9 g/dl* |
| Severe bleed | History of collapse **and/or** Shock<br>■ Systolic BP <100 mmHg<br>■ Pulse >100/min | ■ Replace fluid rapidly<br>■ Ensure blood is available<br>■ Transfuse red cells according to clinical assessment and Hb/Hct | ■ Maintain urine output >0.5 ml/kg/hour<br>■ Maintain systolic BP >100 mmHg<br>■ Maintain Hb >9 g/dl* |

* Until you are confident that the patient is not likely to have a further large bleed. The patient may need to be referred for surgical intervention, once resuscitated.

**Notes**

# Obstetrics

## Key points

1 Anaemia in pregnancy is a haemoglobin concentration of less than 11 g/dl in the first and third trimesters and 10.5 g/dl in the second trimester.

2 The diagnosis and effective treatment of chronic anaemia in pregnancy is an important way of reducing the need for future transfusions. The decision to transfuse blood should not be based on haemoglobin levels alone, but also on the patient's clinical need.

3 Blood loss during normal vaginal delivery or Caesarean section does not normally necessitate transfusion provided that the maternal haemoglobin is above 10.0–11.0 g/dl before delivery.

4 Obstetric bleeding may be unpredictable and massive. Every obstetric unit should have a current protocol for major obstetric haemorrhage and all staff should be trained to follow it.

5 If disseminated intravascular coagulation is suspected, do not delay treatment while waiting for the results of coagulation tests.

6 The administration of anti-RhD immunoglobulin to all RhD negative mothers within 72 hours of delivery is the most common approach to the prevention of haemolytic disease of the newborn.

# Haematological changes in pregnancy

The following haematological changes occur during pregnancy:

- 40–50% increase in plasma volume, reaching its maximum by week 32 of gestation, with similar increase in cardiac output
- Increase in red cell volume by approximately 18–25%, though more slowly than the increase in plasma volume
- Natural reduction in haemoglobin concentration: normal or elevated haemoglobin may signify pre-eclampsia in which plasma volume is reduced
- Increased iron requirement, particularly in last trimester
- Increases in platelet activation and levels of coagulation factors, particularly fibrinogen, Factor VIII and Factor IX
- Fibrinolytic system is suppressed
- Increased susceptibility to thromboembolism.

## Blood loss during delivery

- About 200 ml of blood during normal vaginal delivery
- Up to 500 ml during Caesarean section.

**This blood loss rarely necessitates transfusion provided that the maternal haemoglobin is above 10.0–11.0 g/dl before delivery.**

Further investigation is needed if haemoglobin concentration does not return to normal by 8 weeks postpartum

# Anaemia in pregnancy

| Stage of pregnancy | Anaemic if less than: (g/dl) |
|---|---|
| First trimester: 0–12 weeks | 11.0 |
| Second trimester: 13–28 weeks | 10.5 |
| Third trimester: 29 weeks–term | 11.0 |

Pregnant women are at special risk of anaemia due to:

- Increased iron requirement during pregnancy
- Short birth intervals (blood loss)
- Prolonged lactation (iron loss).

Especially when combined with:

- Parasitic and helminthic infestation
- Malaria
- Sickle cell disease
- HIV infection.

Leading to:

- Iron deficiency
- Folate deficiency.

## Prevention of anaemia in pregnancy

The need for transfusion can often be avoided by the prevention of anaemia through:

- Education about nutrition, food preparation and breastfeeding
- Adequate maternal and child health care
- Access to family planning information, education and services
- Clean water supplies
- Adequate facilities for the disposal of human waste.

Prophylactic administration of iron and folic acid is strongly indicated during pregnancy in countries where iron and folate deficiency is common. Examples of the dose regime are:

1  Optimum daily doses to prevent nutritional anaemia in pregnant women:
   - 120 mg elemental iron
   - 1 mg folate.

2  When anaemia is already present, especially if severe, higher daily therapeutic doses may be more effective:
   - 180 mg elemental iron
   - 2 mg folate.

## Clinical assessment

When anaemia is detected, it is important to determine the cause and assess its severity, including any evidence of clinical decompensation.

Assessment should be based on:

- Patient's clinical history
- Physical examination
- Laboratory investigations to determine the specific cause of anaemia: e.g. serum $B_{12}$, folate or ferritin.

## HISTORY

### Non-specific symptoms of anaemia

- Tiredness/loss of energy
- Light-headedness
- Shortness of breath
- Ankle swelling
- Headache
- Worsening of any pre-existing symptoms: e.g. angina

### History and symptoms relating to the underlying disorder

- Nutritional deficiency: poor dietary history
- Short birth intervals
- Previous history of anaemia

### Bleeding during current pregnancy

## PHYSICAL EXAMINATION

### Signs of anaemia and clinical decompensation

- Pale mucous membranes (palms, nail-beds)
- Rapid breathing
- Tachycardia
- Raised jugular venous pressure
- Heart murmurs
- Ankle oedema
- Postural hypotension
- Altered mental state

### Signs of the underlying disorder (see p. 89)

### Evidence of blood loss

## Transfusion

The decision to transfuse blood should not be based on haemoglobin levels alone, but also on the patient's clinical need.

The following factors must be taken into account:

- Stage of pregnancy (see p. 126)
- Evidence of cardiac failure
- Presence of infection: e.g. pneumonia, malaria
- Obstetric history
- Anticipated delivery:
  — Vaginal
  — Caesarean section
- Haemoglobin level.

## EXAMPLE OF TRANSFUSION GUIDELINES FOR CHRONIC ANAEMIA IN PREGNANCY

### Duration of pregnancy less than 36 weeks

1  Haemoglobin 5.0 g/dl or below, even without clinical signs of cardiac failure or hypoxia.

2  Haemoglobin between 5.0 and 7.0 g/dl and in the presence of the following conditions:
   - Established or incipient cardiac failure or clinical evidence of hypoxia
   - Pneumonia or any other serious bacterial infection
   - Malaria
   - Pre-existing heart disease, not causally related to the anaemia.

### Duration of pregnancy 36 weeks or more

1  Haemoglobin 6.0 g/dl or below.

2  Haemoglobin between 6.0 g/dl and 8.0 g/dl and in the presence of the following conditions:
   - Established or incipient cardiac failure or clinical evidence of hypoxia
   - Pneumonia or any other serious bacterial infection
   - Malaria
   - Pre-existing heart disease, not causally related to the anaemia.

### Elective Caesarean section

When elective Caesarean section is planned and there is a history of:
   - Antepartum haemorrhage (APH)
   - Postpartum haemorrhage (PPH)
   - Previous Caesarean section.

1  Haemoglobin between 8.0 and 10.0 g/dl: establish/confirm blood group and save freshly taken serum for crossmatching.

2  Haemoglobin less than 8.0 g/dl: two units of blood should be crossmatched and available.

### Note

These guidelines are simply an example. Specific indications for transfusion for chronic anaemia in pregnancy should be developed locally.

**Transfusion does not treat the cause of anaemia or correct the non-haematological effects of iron deficiency.**

# Major obstetric haemorrhage

Acute blood loss is one of the main causes of maternal mortality. It may be a result of excessive bleeding from the placental site, trauma to the genital tract and adjacent structures, or both. Increasing parity increases the incidence of obstetric haemorrhage.

Serious haemorrhage may occur at any time throughout pregnancy and the puerperium. See p. 128 for clinical conditions in which there is a risk of acute blood loss.

Major obstetric haemorrhage can be defined as any blood loss occurring in the peripartum period, revealed or concealed, that is likely to endanger life.

**At term, blood flow to the placenta is approximately 700 ml per minute. The patient's entire blood volume can be lost in 5–10 minutes. Unless the myometrium contracts on the placental site appropriately, rapid blood loss will continue, even after the third stage of labour is complete.**

- Obstetric bleeding may be unpredictable and massive
- Major obstetric haemorrhage may result in clear signs of hypovolaemic shock **but**
- Because of the physiological changes induced by pregnancy, there may be few signs of hypovolaemia, despite considerable blood loss.

### Signs of hypovolaemia

- Tachypnoea
- Thirst
- Hypotension
- Tachycardia
- Increased capillary refill time
- Reduced urine output
- Decreased conscious level

It is essential to monitor and investigate a patient with an obstetric haemorrhage, even in the absence of signs of hypovolaemic shock. Be ready and prepared to resuscitate, if necessary.

## CAUSES OF ACUTE BLOOD LOSS IN THE OBSTETRIC PATIENT

| | |
|---|---|
| Fetal loss in pregnancy | ■ Incomplete abortion<br>■ Septic abortion |
| Ectopic pregnancy | ■ Tubal<br>■ Abdominal |
| Antepartum haemorrhage | ■ Placenta praevia<br>■ Abruptio placentae<br>■ Ruptured uterus<br>■ Vasa praevia<br>■ Incidental haemorrhage from cervix or vagina |
| Traumatic lesions, including: | ■ Episiotomy<br>■ Laceration of perineum or vagina<br>■ Laceration of cervix<br>■ Ruptured uterus |
| Primary postpartum haemorrhage (PPH): haemorrhage in excess of 500 ml from genital tract, within 24 hours of delivery | ■ Uterine atony<br>■ Retained products of conception<br>■ Traumatic lesions<br>■ Abnormally adherent placenta: e.g. placenta accreta<br>■ Clotting defects<br>■ Acute uterine inversion |
| Secondary postpartum haemorrhage: any haemorrhage from genital tract, after 24 hours and within 6 weeks of delivery | ■ Puerperal sepsis<br>■ Retained products of conception<br>■ Tissue damage following obstructed labour<br>■ Breakdown of uterine wound after Caesarean section |
| Disseminated intravascular coagulation (DIC) induced by: | ■ Intrauterine death<br>■ Amniotic fluid embolism<br>■ Sepsis<br>■ Pre-eclampsia<br>■ Abruptio placentae<br>■ Retained products of conception<br>■ Induced abortion<br>■ Excessive bleeding<br>■ Acute fatty liver |

## MANAGEMENT OF MAJOR OBSTETRIC HAEMORRHAGE

### RESUSCITATE

1 Administer high concentrations of oxygen.

2 Head down tilt/raise legs.

3 Establish intravenous access with 2 large-bore cannulae (14 g or 16 g).

4 Infuse crystalloid replacement fluids or colloids as rapidly as possible. Restoration of normovolaemia is a priority.

5 Inform blood bank this is an emergency.

Give group O negative antibody-screened blood, and/or uncrossmatched group specific blood until fully crossmatched blood is available.

In areas where the population contains extremely low numbers of women who are RhD negative, use group O blood.

6 Use a pressure infusion device and warming device, if possible.

7 Call extra staff to help:
- Senior obstetrician
- Senior anaesthetist
- Midwives
- Nurses
- Alert the haematologist (if one is available)
- Ensure assistants are available at short notice.

### MONITOR/INVESTIGATE

1 Send sample to blood bank for crossmatching of further blood, but do not wait for crossmatched blood if there is serious haemorrhage.

2 Order full blood count.

3 Order coagulation screen.

4 Continuously monitor pulse rate and blood pressure.

5 Insert urinary catheter and measure hourly output.

6 Monitor respiratory rate.

7 Monitor conscious level.

8 Monitor capillary refill time.

9 Insert central venous pressure line, if available, and monitor CVP.

10 Continue to monitor haemoglobin or haematocrit.

| MANAGEMENT OF MAJOR OBSTETRIC HAEMORRHAGE (continued) |
| --- |

**STOP THE BLEEDING**

1 Identify the cause.

2 Examine cervix and vagina for lacerations.

3 If retained products of conception and uncontrolled bleeding, treat as disseminated intravascular coagulation.

4 If uterus hypotonic and atonic:
   - Ensure bladder is empty
   - Give IV oxytocin 20 units
   - Give IV ergometrine 0.5 mg
   - Oxytocin infusion (40 units in 500 ml)
   - 'Rub up' fundus to stimulate a contraction
   - Bi-manual compression of the uterus (see below)
   - If bleeding continues, deep intramuscular or intramyometrial prostaglandin (e.g. Carboprost 250 mg) directly into uterus (dilute 1 ampoule in 10 ml sterile saline).

5 Consider surgery earlier rather than later.

6 Consider hysterectomy earlier rather than later.

**Bi-manual compression of the uterus**

Press the fingers of one hand into the anterior fornix. The whole fist can be inserted if a good pressure is not obtained as the vagina is lax.

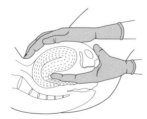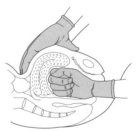

# Disseminated intravascular coagulation

In disseminated intravascular coagulation (DIC), the coagulation and fibrinolytic systems are both activated, leading to deficiencies of the coagulation factors, fibrinogen and platelets. In obstetrics, DIC is a cause of massive haemorrhage. See p. 128 for causes.

**If DIC is suspected, do not delay treatment while waiting for the results of coagulation tests.**

---

## MANAGEMENT OF DISSEMINATED INTRAVASCULAR COAGULATION

See pp. 115–117.

1 Treat the cause:
   - Deliver fetus and placenta
   - Evacuate uterus, as indicated for retained or necrotic tissue.

2 Give uterine stimulants to promote contraction: e.g. oxytocin, ergometrine and/or prostaglandin.

3 Use blood products to help control haemorrhage. In many cases of acute blood loss, the development of DIC can be prevented if blood volume is restored with a balanced salt solution: e.g. Hartmann's solution or Ringer's lactate.

   If needed for oxygen perfusion, give the freshest whole blood available (or packed red cells).

4 Avoid the use of cryoprecipitate and platelet concentrates unless bleeding is uncontrollable.

   If bleeding is not controlled and if coagulation tests show very low platelets, fibrinogen, prolonged PT or APTT, replace coagulation factors and platelets with:
   - Cryoprecipitate: at least 15 packs, prepared from single donor units, containing 3–4 gm fibrinogen in total.

   If cryoprecipitate is not available, give:
   - Fresh frozen plasma (15 ml/kg): 1 unit for every 4–6 units of blood to prevent coagulation defects resulting from use of stored red cell concentrates/suspensions.

   If there is thrombocytopenia, give:
   - Platelet concentrates: rarely necessary to control obstetric haemorrhage with DIC in a woman with previously normal platelet production.

   If these blood components are not available, give the freshest whole blood available (ideally no more than 36 hours old).

5 Give broad spectrum antibiotics, as indicated, to cover aerobic and anaerobic organisms.

# Haemolytic disease of the newborn (HDN)

Haemolytic disease of the newborn is caused by antibodies that are produced by the mother. These antibodies are IgG and can cross the placenta and destroy the baby's red cells. The mother may develop these antibodies:

- If fetal red blood cells cross the placenta (feto-maternal haemorrhage) during pregnancy or delivery
- As a result of a previous transfusion.

HDN due to ABO incompatibility between mother and infant does not affect the fetus *in utero*, but is an important cause of neonatal jaundice.

HDN due to RhD incompatibility is an important cause of severe fetal anaemia in countries where a significant proportion of the population is RhD negative. RhD-negative mothers develop antibodies to an RhD-positive fetus, especially when the mother and infant are of the same or compatible ABO blood type. The fetal red cells are haemolysed, causing severe anaemia.

In the most severe cases of HDN:

- The fetus may die *in utero*
- The fetus may be born with severe anaemia that requires replacement of red cells by exchange transfusion
- There may also be severe neurological damage after birth as a result of a high bilirubin level unless this is corrected by exchange transfusion (see pp. 147–153).

HDN due to other blood group antibodies can also occur, in particular anti-c (also within the Rh blood group system) and anti-Kell. With some very rare exceptions, these two antibodies together with anti-D are the only ones likely to cause significant anaemia *in utero* requiring fetal transfusion.

## Screening in pregnancy

1 The ABO and RhD group of all pregnant women should be determined when they first attend for antenatal care. The mother's blood should also be tested for any IgG antibodies to red cells that can cause HDN.

2 If no antibodies are detected at the first antenatal visit, the pregnant woman should have a further antibody check at 28–30 weeks gestation.

3  If antibodies are detected at the first antenatal visit, the levels should be monitored frequently throughout the pregnancy in case they increase. Rising levels are likely to be indicative of HDN developing in the fetus. Amniocentesis and the level of bilirubin in the amniotic fluid will give a clearer guide to the severity of the disease.

## Anti-RhD immunoglobulin

Anti-RhD immunoglobulin prevents the sensitization and production of antibodies in an RhD negative mother to RhD positive red cells that may have entered the maternal circulation.

### Postpartum prophylaxis

Postpartum prophylaxis is the most common approach to the prevention of haemolytic disease of the newborn.

1  Give anti-RhD immunoglobulin in a dose of 500 mg/IM to an RhD negative mother within 72 hours of delivery if the fetus is RhD positive.

This gives protection for up to 4 ml of fetal red cells.

2  Give further anti-RhD immunoglobulin in a dose of 125 mg/ 1.0 ml of fetal red cells if the Kleihauer or other test is performed and shows more than 4 ml of fetal red cells in the maternal circulation.

### Selective prophylaxis

If any sensitizing event (see p. 134) occurs during the antenatal period, give:

1  250 mg of anti-RhD immunoglobulin up to 20 weeks gestation.

2  500 mg of anti-RhD immunoglobulin from 20 weeks to term.

### Antenatal prophylaxis

Some countries now recommend that all pregnant women who are RhD negative should receive routine anti-RhD immunoglobulin prophylaxis.

There are two options for an intramuscular dosage schedule, both of which appear equally effective:

1  500 mg at 28 and 34 weeks.

2  Single larger dose: 1,200 mg early in the third trimester.

## SELECTIVE PROPHYLAXIS IN THE ANTENATAL PERIOD

- Procedures during pregnancy:
    - Amniocentesis
    - Cordocentesis
    - Chorionic villus blood sampling
- Threatened abortion
- Abortion (particularly therapeutic abortion)
- Antepartum haemorrhage (placenta praevia, abruptio placentae)
- Abdominal trauma
- External cephalic version
- Fetal death
- Multiple pregnancy
- Caesarean section
- Ectopic pregnancy

**Notes**

# Paediatrics & neonatology

## Key points

1 The prevention and early treatment of anaemia is a vital part of the strategy to reduce the need for paediatric transfusion.

2 If hypoxia occurs despite the normal compensatory responses to anaemia, immediate supportive care is required. If the child continues to be clinically unstable, a transfusion may be indicated.

3 The decision to transfuse should not be based on the haemoglobin level alone, but also on a careful assessment of the child's clinical condition.

4 In patients at risk of circulatory overload, transfusion of red cells is preferable to whole blood. Paediatric blood packs should be used, if available, to decrease exposure to multiple donors.

5 In some conditions, such as haemoglobinopathies (sickle cell disease and thalassaemia) repeated red cell transfusions may be indicated.

6 There are very few indications for transfusing fresh frozen plasma. Inappropriate and ineffective use can transmit infectious agents and should be avoided.

# Paediatric anaemia

Paediatric anaemia is defined as a reduction of haemoglobin concentration or red cell blood volume below the normal values for healthy children. Normal haemoglobin/haematocrit values differ according to the child's age.

| Age | Haemoglobin concentration (g/dl) |
|---|---|
| Cord blood (term) | ± 16.5 g/dl |
| Neonate: Day 1 | ± 18.0 g/dl |
| 1 month | ± 14.0 g/dl |
| 3 months | ± 11.0 g/dl |
| 6 months–6 years | ± 12.0 g/dl |
| 7–13 years | ± 13.0 g/dl |
| > 14 years | Same as adults, by sex |

## Causes

Very young children are at particular risk of severe anaemia. The majority of paediatric transfusions are given to children under three years of age. This is due to a combination of the following factors occurring during a rapid growth phase when blood volume is expanding:

- Iron-poor weaning diets
- Recurrent or chronic infection
- Haemolytic episodes in malarious areas.

**A severely anaemic child with other illness (e.g. acute infection), has a high risk of mortality. As well as treating the anaemia, it is essential to look for and treat other conditions: e.g. diarrhoeal disease, pneumonia and malaria.**

## Prevention

The most effective and cost-effective means of preventing anaemia-associated mortality and the use of blood transfusion is to prevent severe anaemia by:

- Early detection of anaemia
- Effective treatment and prophylaxis of the underlying causes of anaemia
- Clinical monitoring of children with mild and moderate anaemia.

**CAUSES OF PAEDIATRIC ANAEMIA**

**Decreased production of normal red blood cells**

- Nutritional deficiencies due to insufficient intake or absorption (iron, $B_{12}$, folate)
- HIV infection
- Chronic disease or inflammation
- Lead poisoning
- Chronic renal disease
- Neoplastic diseases (leukaemia, neoplasms invading bone marrow)

**Increased destruction of red blood cells**

- Malaria
- Haemoglobinopathies (sickle cell disease, thalassaemia)
- G6PD deficiency
- RhD or ABO incompatibility in the newborn
- Autoimmune disorders
- Spherocytosis

**Loss of red blood cells**

- Hookworm infection
- Acute trauma
- Surgery
- Repeated diagnostic blood sampling

## Clinical assessment

Clinical assessment of the degree of anaemia should be supported by a reliable determination of haemoglobin or haematocrit.

Prompt recognition and treatment of malaria (see pp. 95–97) and any associated complications can be life-saving since death can occur within 48 hours.

## Management of compensated anaemia

In children, as in adults, the body's mechanisms to compensate for chronic anaemia often mean that very low haemoglobin levels can be tolerated with few or no symptoms, provided anaemia develops slowly over weeks or months.

A child with well-compensated anaemia may have:

- Raised respiratory rate
- Increased heart rate.

But will be:

- Alert
- Able to drink or breastfeed
- Normal, quiet breathing, with abdominal movement
- Minimal chest movement.

## Management of decompensated anaemia

Many factors can precipitate decompensation in an anaemic child and lead to life-threatening hypoxia of tissues and organs.

### Causes of decompensation

1. Increased demand for oxygen:
   - Infection
   - Pain
   - Fever
   - Exercise.

2. Further reduction in oxygen supply
   - Acute blood loss
   - Pneumonia.

### Early signs of decompensation

- Laboured, rapid breathing with intercostal, subcostal and suprasternal retraction/recession (respiratory distress)
- Increased use of abdominal muscles for breathing
- Flaring of nostrils
- Difficulty with feeding.

### Signs of acute decompensation

- Forced expiration ('grunting')/respiratory distress
- Mental status changes
- Diminished peripheral pulses
- Congestive cardiac failure
- Hepatomegaly
- Poor peripheral perfusion (capillary refill time greater than 2 seconds).

### Supportive treatment

Immediate supportive treatment is needed if the child is severely anaemic with:

- Respiratory distress
- Difficulty in feeding
- Congestive cardiac failure
- Mental status changes.

---

**A child with these clinical signs needs urgent treatment as there is a high risk of death due to insufficient oxygen-carrying capacity.**

---

#### MANAGEMENT OF SEVERE DECOMPENSATED ANAEMIA

1. Position the child and airway to improve ventilation: e.g. sitting up.

2. Give high concentrations of oxygen to improve oxygenation.

3. Take blood sample for crossmatching, haemoglobin estimation and other relevant tests.

4. Control temperature or fever to reduce oxygen demands:
   - Cool by tepid sponging
   - Give antipyretics: e.g. paracetamol.

5. Treat volume overload and cardiac failure with diuretics: e.g. frusemide, 2 mg/kg orally or 1 mg/kg intravenously to a maximum dose of 20 mg/24 hours.

   The dose may need to be repeated if signs of cardiac failure persist.

6. Treat acute bacterial infection or malaria.

#### REASSESSMENT

1. Reassess before giving blood as children often stabilize with diuretics, positioning and oxygen.

2. Clinically assess the need to increase oxygen-carrying capacity.

3. Check haemoglobin concentration to determine severity of anaemia.

---

Severely anaemic children are, contrary to common belief, rarely in congestive heart failure, and dyspnoea is due to acidosis. The sicker the child, the more rapidly transfusion needs to be started.

# Transfusion

**The decision to transfuse should not be based on the haemoglobin level alone, but also on a careful assessment of the child's clinical condition.**

Both laboratory and clinical assessment are essential. A child with moderate anaemia and pneumonia may have more need of increased oxygen-carrying capacity than one with a lower haemoglobin level who is clinically stable.

If the child is stable, is monitored closely and is treated effectively for other conditions, such as acute infection, oxygenation may improve without the need for transfusion.

### INDICATIONS FOR TRANSFUSION

1 Haemoglobin concentration of 4 g/dl or less (or haematocrit 12%), whatever the clinical condition of the patient.

2 Haemoglobin concentration of 4–6 g/dl (or haematocrit 13–18%) if any of the following clinical features are present:
- Clinical features of hypoxia:
  — Acidosis (usually causes dyspnoea)
  — Impaired consciousness
- Hyperparasitaemia (>20%).

The procedure for paediatric transfusion is shown on p. 142.

## Special equipment for paediatric and neonatal transfusion

**Never re-use an adult unit of blood for a second paediatric patient because of the risk of bacteria entering the pack during the first transfusion and proliferating while the blood is out of the refrigerator.**

- Where possible, use paediatric blood packs which enable repeat transfusions to be given to the same patient from a single donation unit; this reduces the risk of infection
- Infants and children require small volumes of fluid and can easily suffer circulatory overload if the infusion is not well-controlled. If possible, use an infusion device that makes it easy to control the rate and volume of infusion.

## TRANSFUSION PROCEDURE

1  If transfusion is needed, give sufficient blood to make the child clinically stable.

2  5 ml/kg of red cells or 10 ml/kg whole blood are usually sufficient to relieve acute shortage of oxygen-carrying capacity. This will increase haemoglobin concentration by approximately 2–3 g/dl unless there is continued bleeding or haemolysis.

3  A red cell transfusion is preferable to whole blood for a patient at risk of circulatory overload, which may precipitate or worsen cardiac failure. 5 ml/kg of red cells gives the same oxygen-carrying capacity as 10 ml/kg of whole blood and contains less plasma protein and fluid to overload the circulation.

4  Where possible, use a paediatric blood pack and a device to control the rate and volume of transfusion.

5  Although rapid fluid infusion increases the risk of volume overload and cardiac failure, give the first 5 ml/kg of red cells to relieve the acute signs of tissue hypoxia. Subsequent transfusion should be given slowly: e.g. 5 ml/kg of red cells over 1 hour.

6  Give frusemide 1 mg/kg orally or 0.5 mg/kg by slow IV injection to a maximum dose of 20 mg/kg if patient is likely to develop cardiac failure and pulmonary oedema. Do not inject it into the blood pack.

7  Monitor during transfusion for signs of:
   - Cardiac failure
   - Fever
   - Respiratory distress
   - Tachypnoea
   - Hypotension
   - Acute transfusion reactions
   - Shock
   - Haemolysis (jaundice, hepatosplenomegaly)
   - Bleeding due to DIC.

8  Re-evaluate the patient's haemoglobin or haematocrit and clinical condition after transfusion.

9  If the patient is still anaemic with clinical signs of hypoxia or a critically low haemoglobin level, give a second transfusion of 5–10 ml/kg of red cells or 10–15 ml/kg of whole blood.

10 Continue treatment of anaemia to help haematological recovery.

# Transfusion in special clinical situations

## Sickle cell disease

- Children with sickle cell disease do not develop symptoms until they are six months old. Transfusions are not necessary to correct the haemoglobin concentration.

- Beyond six months, sicklers have long periods of well-being, punctuated by crises. The main aim of management is to prevent sickle crises.

- Exchange transfusion is indicated for treatment of vaso-occlusive crisis and priapism that does not respond to fluid therapy alone (see p. 149 for calculations for exchange transfusion).

### PREVENTION OF SICKLE CRISIS

1 Give life-time prophylaxis of bacterial infection:

| Oral penicillin V | Year 1 | 62.5 mg/day |
|---|---|---|
| | 1–3 years | 125 mg/day |
| | >3 years | 250 mg/day |

2 Vaccinate against *pneumococcal* infection.

3 Treat infection early.

4 Give folic acid: 1–5 mg/day.

4 Maintain hydration by oral, nasogastric or intravenous fluids during episodes of vomiting and/or diarrhoea.

### TREATMENT OF SICKLE CRISIS

1 Maintain hydration by oral, nasogastric or intravenous fluids.

2 Give supplementary oxygen by mask to maintain adequate oxygenation.

3 Give prompt and effective pain relief.

4 Give antibiotics:
- If causative organism is not identified, give a broad-spectrum antibiotic: e.g. amoxicyllin 125–500 mg/3 times/day
- If causative organism is identified, give the most specific antibiotic available.

5 Transfusion or exchange transfusion.

## Thalassaemia

- Children with more severe forms of thalassaemia cannot maintain oxygenation of tissues and the haemoglobin has to be corrected by regular transfusion
- Iron overload can only be prevented by regular treatment with chelating agents such as desferrioxamine, the most efficient, which has to be given parenterally (see p. 108).

## Malignant disorders

- Leukaemia and other malignancies can cause anaemia and thrombocytopenia
- If a child needs repeated transfusions after a period of months, consider the diagnosis of a malignancy; a full blood count is the first essential laboratory test
- Treatment with chemotherapy often causes severe anaemia and thrombocytopenia. These infants may need repeated blood and platelet transfusions for several weeks during and after chemotherapy until bone marrow recovery occurs.

## Bleeding and clotting disorders

- Disorders of haemostasis should be suspected in a child with a history of bleeding problems.
- Children with coagulation problems (such as haemophilia) may have:
  — Episodes of internal bleeding into joints and muscles
  — Large bruises and haematomas.
- Children with low platelet counts or defective platelet function are more likely to have:
  — Petechiae
  — Multiple small bruises (ecchymoses)
  — Mucous membrane bleeding (mouth, nose, gastro-intestinal).

## Congenital disorders

See pp. 109–114 for haemophilia A, haemophilia B and von Willebrand's disease.

## Acquired disorders

### Vitamin K deficiency in the neonate

- A transient decrease in vitamin K-dependent coagulation factors (II, VII, IX, X) occurs normally in the neonate 48–72 hours after birth
- There is a gradual return to normal levels by 7–10 days of age
- Prophylactic IM administration of 1 mg of oil-soluble vitamin K at birth prevents haemorrhagic disease of the newborn in full-term and most premature infants.

Despite prophylaxis, some premature infants and some full-term newborns may develop haemorrhagic disease of the newborn:

- Infants of mothers taking anticonvulsant drugs (phenobarbitol and phenytoin) are at increased risk
- An affected infant has a prolonged PT and APTT, while platelets and fibrinogen levels are normal
- Treat bleeding as a result of deficiencies of vitamin K-dependent coagulation factors with 1–5 mg vitamin K intravenously
- Transfusion of fresh frozen plasma may be required to clinically correct a significant bleeding tendency
- Late onset disease (more than one week after birth) is often associated with malabsorption of vitamin K. This may be due to intestinal malabsorption and liver disease. It can be treated with oral water-soluble vitamin K.

## Thrombocytopenia

- A normal neonate's platelet count is $80–450 \times 10^9$/L
- After one week of age, it reaches adult levels of $150–400 \times 10^9$/L
- Platelet counts below this level are considered to be thrombocytopenia.

The patient with thrombocytopenia due to bleeding typically has:

- Petechiae
- Retinal haemorrhages
- Bleeding gums
- Bleeding from venepuncture sites.

## Management

The treatment of thrombocytopenia varies according to the cause:

- Idiopathic thrombocytopenic purpura is usually self-limited, but may be treated with immunoglobulin and corticosteroids; blood or platelet transfusion may be indicated if life-threatening haemorrhage occurs

- Other acquired disorders should be managed with supportive care, treatment of infection and stopping drugs that may be causing the disorder

- Immune neonatal thrombocytopenia: intravenous immuno-globulin may be helpful. If available, the transfusion of compatible platelets (e.g. washed and irradiated platelets collected from the infant's mother) is effective.

### Platelet transfusion for bleeding due to thrombocytopenia

The goal of platelet therapy is to control or stop the bleeding. The clinical response is more important than the platelet count.

---

#### TRANSFUSION OF PLATELET CONCENTRATES

**Dose units**: Platelet concentrate from 1 donor unit (450 ml) of whole blood contains about 60 x $10^9$/L

| Dosage | | Volume | Platelet concentrate |
|---|---|---|---|
| Up to 15 kg | 1 platelet concentrate | 30–50 ml* | 60 x $10^9$/L |
| 15–30 kg | 2 platelet concentrate | 60–100 ml | 120 x $10^9$/L |
| >30 kg | 4 platelet concentrate | 120–400 ml | 240 x $10^9$/L |

\* For small infants, the blood bank may remove part of the plasma before transfusion

#### ADMINISTRATION OF PLATELET CONCENTRATES

1 Transfuse immediately on receiving the platelet concentrates.

2 Do not refrigerate.

3 Use a fresh, standard blood infusion set, primed with normal saline.

---

### Prophylactic platelet transfusion

- Indicated in a stable thrombocytopenic patient without evidence of bleeding, when the platelet count falls below 10 x $10^9$/L

- Some clinicians favour a higher threshold of between 10–20 x $10^9$/L in a patient who is stable
- If the patient is feverish or infected, a threshold of 20–50 x $10^9$/L may be appropriate.

## Neonatal transfusion

### SELECTING PRODUCTS FOR NEONATAL TRANSFUSION

| Product | Indication | Special requirements |
|---|---|---|
| Whole blood | Exchange transfusions for HDN | Freshest blood available (less than 5 days after collection), free of relevant alloantibodies |
| Red cells | 'Top-up' transfusion to raise haemoglobin concentration in symptomatic chronic anaemia, often due to blood sampling in sick premature infants | Small dose units (paediatric packs from a single donation) to minimize exposure to different donors |
| Specially-processed cellular components | Intrauterine transfusion:<br>■ Risk of GvHD may be greater in premature infants<br>■ Risk of GvHD is greater if donor is a blood relative | Avoid graft-versus-host disease:<br>■ Irradiate: 25 Gy<br>■ Do not use donation from blood relative |
| CMV-negative donations<br>*and/or*<br>Leucocyte-depleted component | CMV infection or reactivation may complicate the management of sick infants. CMV may be transmitted by blood or infection reactivated by allogenic leucocyte transfusion | Avoid CMV infection in recipient |

### Exchange transfusion

- The main indication for neonatal exchange transfusion is to prevent neurological complications (kernicterus) caused by a rapidly-rising unconjugated bilirubin concentration

- This occurs because the immature liver cannot metabolise the breakdown products of haemoglobin. The underlying cause is usually haemolysis (red cell destruction) due to antibodies to the neonatal red blood cells.

If exchange transfusion is needed:

1 Use a group O blood unit that does not carry the antigen against which the maternal antibody is directed:
   - For HDN due to anti-D: use group O RhD negative
   - For HDN due to anti-Rh c: use group O RhD positive that does not have the c antigen ($R_1R_1$, CDe/CDe).

2 An exchange transfusion of about two times the neonate's blood volume (about 170 ml/kg) is most effective to reduce bilirubin and restore the haemoglobin level; this can usually be carried out with one unit of whole blood.

3 A unit of whole donor blood will normally have a haematocrit of 37–45%, which is more than adequate for neonatal needs.

4 There is no need to adjust the haematocrit of the unit: if it is raised to 50–60%, there is a risk of polycythaemia and its consequences, especially if the neonate is also receiving phototherapy.

| Age | Total blood volume |
| --- | --- |
| Premature infants | 100 ml/kg |
| Term newborns | 85–90 ml/kg |
| >1 month | 80 ml/kg |
| >1 year | 70 ml/kg |

Pages 149–151 provide guidelines on calculations and the procedure for neonatal exchange transfusion, precautions and possible complications.

## Haemolytic disease of the newborn due to materno-fetal ABO incompatibility (ABO-HDN)

See also p. 132. In many parts of the world, HDN due to ABO incompatibility is the most important cause of severe neonatal jaundice and is the most frequent indication for exchange transfusion in the newborn.

## CALCULATIONS FOR NEONATAL EXCHANGE TRANSFUSION

### Partial exchange transfusion for treatment of symptomatic polycythaemia

Replace removed blood volume with normal saline or 5% albumin

Volume to be exchanged (ml):

$$\text{Estimated blood volume} \times \frac{\text{(Patient's Hct – Desired Hct)}}{\text{Patient's Hct}}$$

### Two-volume red cell exchange transfusion for treatment of sickle cell crisis and neonatal hyperbilirubinaemia

Replace calculated blood volume with whole blood or red cells suspended in 5% human albumin

Volume to be exchanged (ml):

$$\text{Estimated blood volume} \times \frac{\text{(Patient's Hct (\%)} \times 2)}{\text{Hct of transfused unit (\%)*}}$$

* Haematocrit

| | |
|---|---|
| Whole blood | 35%–45% |
| Red cell concentrate | 55%–75% |
| Red cell suspension | 50%–70% |

## TRANSFUSION PROCEDURE

1 Give nothing by mouth to the infant during and at least 4 hours after exchange transfusion. Empty stomach if the infant was fed within 4 hours of the procedure.

2 Closely monitor vital signs, blood sugar and temperature. Have resuscitation equipment ready.

3 For a newborn, umbilical and venous catheters inserted by sterile technique may be used (blood is drawn out of the arterial catheter and infused through the venous catheter). Alternatively, two peripheral lines may be used.

4 Prewarm blood only if a quality-controlled blood warmer is available. Do *not* improvise by using a waterbath.

5 Exchange 15 ml increments in a full-term infant and smaller volumes for smaller, less stable infants. Do not allow cells in the donor unit to form a sediment.

6   Withdraw and infuse blood 2–3 ml/kg/minute to avoid mechanical trauma to the patient and donor cells.

7   Give 1–2 ml of 10% calcium gluconate solution IV slowly for ECG evidence of hypocalcaemia (prolonged Q-T intervals). Flush tubing with normal saline before and after calcium infusion. Observe for brachycardia during infusion.

8   To complete two-volume exchange, transfuse 170 ml/kg for a full-term infant and 170–200 ml/kg for a pre-term infant.

9   Send the last aliquot drawn to the laboratory for determination of haemoglobin or haematocrit, blood smear, glucose, bilirubin, potassium, calcium, and group and match.

10  Prevent hypoglycaemia after exchange transfusion by continuing infusion of a glucose-containing crystalloid.

## PRECAUTIONS

1   When exchange transfusion is performed to treat haemolytic disease of the newborn, the transfused red cells must be compatible with the mother's serum since the haemolysis is caused by maternal IgG antibodies that cross the placenta and destroy the fetal red cells.

The blood should therefore be crossmatched against the mother's serum using the antiglobulin method that detects IgG antibodies.

2   There is no need to adjust the haematocrit of donor whole blood.

## COMPLICATIONS OF EXCHANGE TRANSFUSION

### Cardiovascular
- Thromboemboli or air emboli
- Portal vein thrombosis
- Dysrhythmias
- Volume overload
- Cardiorespiratory arrest

### Fluid and electrolyte disturbances
- Hyperkalaemia
- Hypernatremia
- Hypocalcaemia
- Hypoglycaemia
- Acidosis

**Haematological**
- Thrombocytopenia
- Disseminated intravascular coagulation
- Over-heparinization (may use 1 mg of protamine per 100 units of heparin in the donor unit)
- Transfusion reaction

**Infection**
- Hepatitis
- HIV
- Sepsis

**Mechanical**
- Injury to donor cells (especially from overheating)
- Injury to vessels
- Blood loss

- The diagnosis of ABO HDN is usually made in infants born at term who are not severely anaemic, but who develop jaundice during the first 24 hours of life

- ABO incompatibility does not present *in utero* and never causes hydrops

- The neonate should receive phototherapy and supportive treatment; treatment should be initiated promptly as jaundice severe enough to lead to kernicterus may develop

- Blood units for exchange transfusion should be group O, with low-titre anti-A and anti-B with no IgG lysins

- A two-volume exchange (approximately 170 ml/kg) is most effective in removing bilirubin

- If the bilirubin rises again to dangerous levels, a further two-volume exchange should be performed.

## Indirect (unconjugated) hyperbilirubinaemia
Healthy term infants may tolerate serum bilirubin levels of 25 mg/dl. Infants are more prone to the toxic effects of bilirubin if they have:
- Acidosis
- Prematurity
- Septicaemia
- Hypoxia

- Hypoglycaemia
- Asphyxia
- Hypothermia
- Hypoproteinaemia
- Exposure to drugs that displace bilirubin from albumin
- Haemolysis.

The goal of therapy is to prevent the concentration of indirect bilirubin from reaching neurotoxic levels.

## SUGGESTED MAXIMUM INDIRECT SERUM BILIRUBIN CONCENTRATIONS (mg/dl) IN PRE-TERM AND TERM INFANTS

| Birthweight (gm) | Uncomplicated | Complicated* |
|---|---|---|
| <1000 | 12–13 | 10–12 |
| 1000–1250 | 12–14 | 10–12 |
| 1251–1499 | 14–16 | 12–14 |
| 1500–1999 | 16–20 | 15–17 |
| >2000/term | 20–22 | 18–20 |

\* Complicated refers to presence of risk factors associated with increased risk of kernicterus, listed above.

## MANAGEMENT OF NEONATES WITH INDIRECT HYPERBILIRUBINAEMIA

1 Treat underlying causes of hyperbilirubinaemia and factors that increase risk of kernicterus (sepsis, hypoxia, etc.).

2 Hydration.

3 Initiate phototherapy at bilirubin levels well below those indicated for exchange transfusion.

   Phototherapy may require 6–12 hours before having a measurable effect.

4 Monitor bilirubin levels in pre-term and term infants.

5 Give exchange transfusion when indirect serum bilirubin levels reach maximum levels.

6 Continue to monitor bilirubin levels until a fall in bilirubin is observed in the absence of phototherapy.

- Exchange transfusion is necessary when:
  — After phototherapy, indirect bilirubin levels approach those considered critical during the first two days of life
  — A further rise is anticipated
- Exchange transfusion may not be necessary after the fourth day in term infants or the seventh day in pre-term infants, when hepatic conjugating mechanisms become more effective and a fall in bilirubin can be anticipated
- An exchange transfusion should be at least one blood volume
- Exchange transfusion should be repeated if the indirect bilirubin level is not maintained at a safe level.

## Partial exchange transfusion

Partial exchange transfusion is often used for treatment of symptomatic polycythaemia and hyperviscosity.

1 Healthy term infants appear to be at little risk of polycythaemia and hyperviscosity and need not be screened routinely.

2 In polycythaemic neonates with mild or no symptoms, keeping the infant warm and well-hydrated is probably all that is required to prevent microthromboses in the peripheral circulation.

3 The generally-accepted screening test is a central venous haematocrit of 65% or more.

4 In infants with suspected hyperviscosity, it is recommended that haematocrit values are measured by microcentrifugation since viscosity tests are unavailable to most physicians.

5 Falsely low values for haematocrit may be given by automated haematology analysers.

All infants with significant symptoms should undergo partial exchange with 4.5% albumin to bring the haematocrit down to a safe level of 50–55%.

---

**CALCULATIONS FOR PARTIAL EXCHANGE TRANSFUSION**

Volume to be exchanged:

$$\text{Estimated blood volume* } \times \frac{(\text{Patient's Hct} - \text{Desired Hct})}{\text{Patient's Hct}}$$

\* Assuming the neonatal blood volume to be 85 ml per kg

1 The volume exchange is usually around 20 ml per kg.

2 The exchange transfusion should be performed in 10 ml aliquots.

---

# Red cell transfusion

The majority of transfusions are given to pre-term infants who are very unwell:

- To replace blood samples taken for laboratory testing
- To treat hypotension and hypovolaemia
- To treat the combined effect of anaemia of prematurity and blood loss due to sampling.

A neonate who requires one blood transfusion will often need to be transfused again within a period of days as neonates do not have an effective erythropoietin response to anaemia.

# Specific clinical situations (neonatal)

### Critically ill neonates

1  Record the volume of each blood sample taken. If 10% of the blood volume is removed over 24–48 hours, it should be replaced with packed red cells.

2  Critically ill neonates may need to have their haemoglobin level maintained in the range of 13–14 g/dl to ensure adequate tissue perfusion.

### Convalescent very low birth weight babies

1  Measure the haemoglobin at weekly intervals. The haemoglobin level will drop 1 g/dl per week on average.

2  Do not transfuse on the basis of the haemoglobin level alone. Although haemoglobin levels of 7 g/dl or less require investigation, transfusion may not be required.

### Neonates with late anaemia

Consider transfusing an infant if anaemia is thought to be the cause of:

1  Poor weight gain.

2  Fatigue while feeding.

3  Tachypnoea and tachycardia.

4  Other signs of decompensation.

# Minimizing the risks and increasing the effective use of neonatal transfusion

The following practical measures reduce the risks of neonatal transfusion and increase its effectiveness.

1 For an infant who is likely to need several 'top-up' transfusions over a period of days or weeks, use red cells in additive solution prepared in paediatric packs from a single unit of blood.

2 Reduce blood loss from diagnostic sampling:
- Avoid unnecessary repeat compatibility testing
- Avoid non-essential laboratory tests
- Where possible, the laboratory should use micro-methods and should select suitable small sample tubes.

3 Avoid transfusing blood donated by blood relatives as the risk of graft-versus-host disease is increased.

## Neonatal alloimmune thrombocytopenia

Neonatal alloimmune thrombocytopenia (NAIT) is a cause of intrauterine cerebral haemorrhage. Transfusion of washed, irradiated platelets may help the infant at a period of dangerous thrombocytopenia.

## Fresh frozen plasma

Fresh frozen plasma should only be used for specific clinical indications for which it is proved to be effective:

- The correction of clinically important bleeding tendencies due to deficiency of plasma clotting factors – and only when a safer, virus-inactivated product is unavailable

- For infusion or exchange transfusion treatment of the rare conditions of thrombotic thrombocytopenic purpura or haemolytic-uraemic syndrome.

**Notes**

# Surgery & anaesthesia

## Key points

1  Most elective surgery does not result in sufficient blood loss to require blood transfusion. There is rarely justification for the use of preoperative blood transfusion simply to facilitate elective surgery.

2  The careful assessment and management of patients prior to surgery will reduce patient morbidity and mortality:
   - Identify and treat anaemia before surgery
   - Identify and treat medical conditions before surgery
   - Identify bleeding disorders and stop medications that impair haemostasis.

3  Minimize operative blood loss by:
   - Meticulous surgical technique
   - Use of posture
   - Use of vasoconstrictors
   - Use of tourniquets
   - Anaesthetic techniques
   - Use of antifibrinolytic drugs.

4  A significant degree of surgical blood loss can often safely be incurred before transfusion becomes necessary, provided that normovolaemia is maintained through the use of intravenous replacement fluids.

5  Use autologous transfusion, where appropriate, to reduce or eliminate the need for transfusion. However, it should only be considered where the surgery is expected to result in sufficient blood loss to require allogeneic transfusion.

6  Blood loss and hypovolaemia can still develop in the postoperative period. Vigilant monitoring of vital signs and the surgical site is an essential part of patient management.

## Transfusion in elective surgery

The use of transfusion for elective surgical procedures varies greatly between hospitals and individual clinicians. These differences are partly due to variations in the medical condition of patients, but are also caused by:

- Differences in surgical and anaesthetic techniques
- Different attitudes to the use of blood
- Differences in the cost and availability of blood products and alternatives to transfusion.

In some patients, the need for transfusion is obvious, but it is often difficult to decide whether transfusion is really necessary.

There is no single, simple measure that shows that oxygenation of the tissues is inadequate or is becoming inadequate. Several factors must be taken into account in assessing the patient, such as:

- Age
- Pre-existing anaemia
- Medical disorders
- Anaesthesia (may mask clinical signs)
- Haemoglobin concentration
- Fluid status.

Many elective surgical procedures rarely require transfusion. However, for some major procedures, blood should be available in advance.

## Preparation of the patient

The careful assessment and management of patients prior to surgery can do much to reduce patient morbidity and mortality. The surgeon who initially assesses the patient must ensure he or she is adequately prepared for surgery and anaesthesia. The anaesthetist should assist the surgeon in that preparation.

Good communication between the surgeon and anaesthetist is vital before, during and after the operation.

### Classification of surgery

Operations are often classed as 'major' or 'minor'. Other factors also influence the likelihood of complications, such as bleeding.

---

**Factors affecting risk of haemorrhage**

---

- Experience of the surgeon or anaesthetist
- Duration of surgery
- Condition of the patient
- Anaesthetic and surgical technique
- Anticipated blood loss

---

# Preoperative anaemia

1 Patients should be tested preoperatively to detect anaemia. Anaemia should be treated and, if possible, its cause diagnosed and treated before planned surgery.

2 In a patient who is already anaemic, a further reduction in oxygen delivery due to acute blood loss or the effects of anaesthetic agents may lead to decompensation.

3 An adequate preoperative haemoglobin level for each patient undergoing elective surgery should be determined, based on the clinical condition of the patient and the nature of the procedure being planned.

4 Ensuring an adequate haemoglobin level before surgery reduces the likelihood of a transfusion being needed if blood loss occurs during surgery. There is rarely justification for the use of preoperative blood transfusion simply to facilitate elective surgery.

## Preoperative haemoglobin level

Many practitioners will accept a threshold haemoglobin level of approximately 7–8 g/dl in a well-compensated and otherwise healthy patient presenting for minor surgery. However, a higher preoperative haemoglobin level will be needed before elective surgery in the following situations.

1 Inadequate compensation for the anaemia.

2 Significant co-existing cardiorespiratory disease.

3 Major surgery or significant blood loss is expected.

## Cardiorespiratory disorders

Co-existing disease processes in a patient, and particularly those affecting the cardiac or respiratory systems, can have a significant influence on oxygen delivery.

Treating and optimizing these disorders preoperatively will:

- Improve the overall oxygen supply to the tissues
- Reduce the possibility of a transfusion becoming necessary at operation.

## Coagulation disorders

Undiagnosed and untreated disorders of coagulation in surgical patients are very likely to result in excessive operative blood loss. They may also lead to uncontrolled haemorrhage and death of the patient.

It is essential to make a careful preoperative enquiry into any unusual bleeding tendency of the patient and his or her family, together with a drug history. If possible, obtain expert haematological advice before surgery in all patients with an established coagulation disorder.

### Surgery and acquired coagulation disorders

Bleeding during or after surgery is sometimes very difficult to evaluate. It may simply be caused by a problem following surgical intervention, in which case re-operation may be necessary. Alternatively, it may be due to any one of a number of haemostatic problems, including:

- Massive transfusion: replacement of blood losses equivalent to or greater than the patient's blood volume in less than 24 hours, leading to dilution of coagulation factors and platelets
- Disseminated intravascular coagulation, which causes:
  — Hypofibrinogenaemia
  — Depletion of coagulation factors
  — Thrombocytopenia.

### Surgery and congenital coagulation disorders

See p. 113 for the prophylactic measures that can be used to allow surgery to be performed safely, depending on the local availability of the various drug and blood products.

Start treatment at least 1–2 days prior to surgery and continue for 5–10 days, depending on the risk of postoperative bleeding. Regular assessment of the patient in the perioperative period is essential to detect unexpected bleeding.

## Thrombocytopenia

A variety of disorders may give rise to a reduced platelet count. Prophylactic measures and the availability of platelet concentrates for transfusion are invariably required for surgery in this group of patients: e.g. splenectomy in a patient with idiopathic thrombocytopenia purpura (ITP).

Platelet transfusions should be given if there is clinical evidence of severe microvascular bleeding and the platelet count is below $50 \times 10^9$/L.

## Anticoagulants: warfarin (coumarin), heparin

In patients who are being treated with anticoagulants (oral or parenteral), the type of surgery and the thrombotic risk should be taken into account when planning anticoagulant control perioperatively.

For most surgical procedures, the INR and/or APTT ratio should be less than 2.0 before surgery commences.

---

**PATIENTS FULLY ANTICOAGULATED WITH WARFARIN**

**Elective surgery**

1  Stop warfarin three days preoperatively and monitor INR daily.

2  Give heparin by infusion or subcutaneously if INR is >2.0.

3  Stop heparin 6 hours preoperatively.

4  Check INR and APTT ratio immediately prior to surgery.

5  Commence surgery if INR and APTT ratio are <2.0.

6  Restart warfarin as soon as possible postoperatively.

7  Restart heparin at the same time and continue until INR is in the therapeutic range.

**Emergency surgery**

1  Give vitamin K, 0.5–2.0 mg by slow IV infusion.

2  Give fresh frozen plasma, 15 ml/kg. This dose may need to be repeated to bring coagulation factors to an acceptable range.

3  Check INR and APTT ratio immediately prior to surgery.

4  Commence surgery if INR and APTT ratio are <2.0.

---

### PATIENTS FULLY ANTICOAGULATED WITH HEPARIN

**Elective surgery**

1   Stop heparin 6 hours preoperatively.

2   Check APTT ratio immediately prior to surgery.

3   Commence surgery if APTT ratio is <2.0.

4   Restart heparin as soon as appropriate postoperatively.

**Emergency surgery**

Consider reversal with IV protamine sulphate. 1 mg of protamine neutralizes 100 iu heparin.

### PATIENTS RECEIVING LOW-DOSE HEPARIN

It is rarely necessary to stop low-dose heparin injections, used in the prevention of deep vein thrombosis and pulmonary embolism, prior to surgery.

## Other drugs and bleeding

Stop drugs that interfere with platelet function (e.g. aspirin and the non-steroidal anti-inflammatory drugs, NSAIDs) 10 days prior to surgery. This can significantly reduce operative blood loss.

# Techniques to reduce operative blood loss

The training, experience and care of the surgeon performing the procedure is the most crucial factor in reducing operative blood loss. The anaesthetist's technique can also greatly influence operative blood loss.

## Surgical technique

1   Attend to bleeding points.

2   Use diathermy, if available.

3   Use local haemostatic: e.g. collagen, fibrin glue or warmed packs.

## Posture of the patient

1   Ensure operative site is slightly above heart level.

2   For lower limb, pelvic and abdominal procedures, use head down (Trendelenburg) position.

3   For head and neck surgery, use the head-up posture.

4   Avoid air embolism if a large vein above heart level is opened during surgery.

## Vasoconstrictors

1   Infiltrate the skin at the site of surgery with a vasoconstrictor to minimize skin bleeding once an incision is made. If the vasoconstrictor also contains local anaesthetic, some contribution to postoperative analgesia can be expected from this technique.

2   Reduce bleeding from skin graft donor sites, desloughed areas and tangential excisions by direct application of swabs soaked in a saline solution containing a vasoconstrictor.

3   Adrenaline (epinephrine) is a widely-used and effective vasoconstrictor. It should not be necessary to exceed a total dose of 0.1 mg in an adult, equivalent to 20 ml of 1 in 200 000 strength or 40 ml of 1 in 400 000 strength.

4   Do not exceed the recommended dose levels of vaso-constrictors and local anaesthetics because of their profound systemic actions. Ensure these drugs remain at the site of incision and are **not** injected into the circulation.

5   Of all the anaesthetic inhalational agents, halothane is the most likely to cause cardiac dysrhythmias when a vaso-constrictor is being used.

6   Do not use vasoconstrictors in areas where there are end arteries: e.g. fingers, toes and penis.

## Tourniquets

1   When operating on extremities, reduce blood loss by the application of a limb tourniquet.

2   Exsanguinate the limb using a bandage or elevation prior to inflation of a suitable-sized, well-fitting tourniquet.

The inflation pressure of the tourniquet should be approximately 100–150 mmHg above the systolic blood pressure of the patient.

3   Towards the end of the procedure, deflate the tourniquet temporarily to identify missed bleeding points and ensure complete haemostasis before finally closing the wound.

4   Do not use tourniquets:
   ■   On patients with sickle cell disease or trait (HbSS, HbAS, HbSC) because of the risk of precipitating sickling
   ■   Where the blood supply to the limb is already tenuous: e.g. severe atherosclerosis.

## Anaesthetic techniques

1   Prevent episodes of hypertension and tachycardia due to sympathetic overactivity by ensuring adequate levels of anaesthesia and analgesia.

2   Avoid coughing, straining and patient manoeuvres that increase venous blood pressure.

3   Control ventilation to avoid excessive carbon dioxide retention, or hypercarbia, which can cause widespread vasodilatation and increase operative blood loss.

4   Use regional anaesthesia, particularly epidural and subarachnoid anaesthetic techniques, to reduce operative blood loss, where appropriate.

5   Do not use hypotensive anaesthesia to reduce operative blood loss where an experienced anaesthetist and comprehensive monitoring facilities are not available.

## Antifibrinolytic and other drugs

Several drugs, including aprotinin and tranexamic acid, which inhibit the fibrinolytic system of blood and encourage clot stability, are used to reduce operative blood loss in cardiac surgery. Wider indications are not yet defined.

Desmopressin (DDAVP) can be effective in preventing excessive bleeding in haemophiliacs and some acquired bleeding disorders, such as cirrhosis of the liver. It acts by increasing the production of Factor VIII.

## Fluid replacement and transfusion

Provided blood volume is maintained with crystalloid or colloid fluids, the patient can often safely tolerate significant blood loss before transfusion of red cells is required, for the following reasons.

1   The supply of oxygen in a healthy, resting adult with a normal haemoglobin concentration is 3–4 times greater than that required by the tissues for metabolism. This safety margin

between oxygen supply and demand allows some reduction in haemoglobin to occur without serious consequences.

2   When significant blood loss occurs, compensatory responses occur that help to maintain the supply of oxygen to the tissues.

3   These compensatory mechanisms are more effective and tissue oxygenation is better preserved If the normal blood volume is maintained by fluid replacement as blood loss occurs. This allows the cardiac output to increase and sustain the oxygen supply if the haemoglobin concentration is falling.

4   The replacement of blood loss with crystalloid or colloid fluids dilutes the blood (haemodilution). This reduces its viscosity and improves both capillary blood flow and cardiac output, enhancing the supply of oxygen to the tissues.

**A key objective is to ensure normovolaemia at all times during the course of a surgical procedure.**

## Estimating blood loss

In order to maintain blood volume accurately, it is essential to continually assess surgical blood loss throughout the procedure. This is especially important in neonatal and infant surgery where only a very small amount lost can represent a significant proportion of blood volume.

| Blood volume | |
|---|---|
| Neonates | 85–90 ml/kg body weight |
| Children | 80 ml/kg body weight |
| Adults | 70 ml/kg body weight |

Example: an adult weighing 60 kg would have a blood volume equal to 70 x 60, which is 4200 ml.

1   Weigh swabs while still in their dry state and in their sterile packs.

2   Weigh the blood-soaked swabs as soon as they are discarded and subtract their dry weight (1 ml of blood weighs approximately 1 g).

3  Weigh ungraduated drains or suction bottles and subtract the empty weight.

4  Estimate blood loss into surgical drapes, together with that pooling beneath the patient and onto the floor.

5  Note the volume of any irrigation or washout fluids that are used during surgery and have contaminated swabs or suction bottles. Subtract this volume from the measured blood loss to arrive at a final estimate.

## Monitoring for signs of hypovolaemia

1  Many of the autonomic and central nervous system signs of significant hypovolaemia can be masked by the effects of general anaesthesia.

2  The classic picture of the restless or confused patient who is hyperventilating (air-hunger), in a cold sweat and complaining of thirst is not a presentation under general anaesthesia.

3  Many of these signs will be apparent in the patient undergoing local or regional anaesthesia and in those recovering from general anaesthesia.

**Patients under a general anaesthetic may show only very few signs that hypovolaemia is developing. Pallor of the mucous membranes, a reduced pulse volume and tachycardia may be the only initial signs.**

### Monitoring for signs of hypovolaemia

- Colour of mucous membranes
- Respiratory rate
- Level of consciousness
- Urine output
- ECG
- CVP, if available and appropriate
- Heart rate
- Capillary refill time
- Blood pressure
- Peripheral temperature
- Saturation of haemoglobin

## Replacement of blood loss

The following methods are commonly used to estimate the volume of surgical blood loss that can be expected (or allowed) to occur in a patient before a blood transfusion becomes necessary.

## PERCENTAGE METHOD OF ESTIMATING ALLOWABLE BLOOD LOSS

This method involves estimating the allowable blood loss as a percentage of the patient's blood volume.

1  Calculate the patient's blood volume.

2  Decide on the percentage of blood volume that could be lost but safely tolerated, provided that normovolaemia is maintained. For example, if 10% were chosen, the allowable blood loss in a 60 kg patient would be 420 ml.

3  During the procedure, replace blood loss up to the allowable volume with crystalloids or colloid fluids to maintain normovolaemia.

4  If the allowable blood loss volume is exceeded, further replacement should be with transfused blood.

## HAEMODILUTION METHOD OF ESTIMATING ALLOWABLE BLOOD LOSS

This method involves estimating the allowable blood loss by judging the lowest haemoglobin (or haematocrit) that could be safely tolerated by the patient as haemodilution with fluid replacement takes place.

1  Calculate the patient's blood volume and perform a preoperative haemoglobin (or haematocrit) level.

2  Decide on the lowest acceptable haemoglobin (or haematocrit) that could be safely tolerated by the patient.

3  Apply the following formula to calculate the allowable volume of blood loss that can occur before a blood transfusion becomes necessary.

$$\text{Allowable loss} = \frac{\text{Blood volume} \times (\text{Preoperative Hb} - \text{Lowest Acceptable Hb})}{(\text{Average of Preoperative \& Lowest Acceptable Hb})}$$

4  During the procedure, replace blood loss up to the allowable volume with crystalloid or colloid fluids to maintain normovolaemia.

5  If the allowable blood loss volume is exceeded, further replacement should be with transfused blood.

These methods are simply guides to fluid replacement and transfusion. During surgery, the decision to transfuse will ultimately need to be based on the careful assessment of:

- Volume of blood loss
- Rate of blood loss (actual and anticipated)

- Patient's clinical response to blood loss and fluid replacement therapy
- Signs indicating inadequate tissue oxygenation.

You must therefore be prepared to move away from any guidelines and transfuse at an earlier stage if the situation warrants it.

---

**It is vital to ensure that either the percentage loss or the lowest acceptable haemoglobin reflect the blood loss that the patient can safely tolerate.**

---

This judgement must be based on the clinical condition of each individual patient. The ability of a patient to compensate for a reduction in oxygen supply will be limited by:

- Evidence of cardiorespiratory disease
- Treatment with drugs such as beta-blockers
- Pre-existing anaemia
- Increasing age.

| METHOD | HEALTHY | AVERAGE CLINICAL CONDITION | POOR CLINICAL CONDITION |
|--------|---------|---------------------------|------------------------|
| **Percentage method** Acceptable loss of blood volume | 30% | 20% | Less than 10% |
| **Haemodilution method** Lowest acceptable haemoglobin (or Hct) | 9 g/dl (Hct 27%) | 10 g/dl (Hct 30%) | 11 g/dl (Hct 33%) |

### Choice of replacement fluid

There continues to be controversy about the choice of fluid used for the initial replacement of blood loss in order to maintain blood volume.

1 Crystalloid replacement fluids, such as normal saline or Ringer's lactate solution, leave the circulation more rapidly than colloids. Use at least three times the volume of blood lost: i.e. 3 ml of crystalloid to every 1 ml of blood loss.

2 If colloid fluids are used, infuse an amount equal to the volume of blood lost.

## Maintaining normovolaemia

It is essential that blood volume is maintained at all times. Even if the allowable blood loss is exceeded and no blood for transfusion is readily available, continue to infuse crystalloid replacement fluids or colloids to ensure normovolaemia.

## Avoiding hypothermia

A fall in body temperature can cause unwanted effects, including:

- Impairment of the normal compensatory responses to hypovolaemia
- Increase in operative bleeding
- Increase in oxygen demand postoperatively as normothermia become re-established; this may lead to hypoxia
- Increase in wound infection.

Maintain a normal body temperature in the perioperative period, including the warming of intravenous fluids. Heat loss occurs more readily in children.

| Patient | Fluids |
| --- | --- |
| ■ Cover with blankets | ■ Store fluids in warming cabinet |
| ■ Use warming mattress (37°C) | ■ Immerse fluid bags in warm water |
| ■ Humidify anaesthetic gases | ■ Use heat exchangers on infusion set |

# Replacement of other fluid losses

Maintain normovolaemia by replacing other fluid losses in addition to blood loss during the operative period.

## Maintenance fluid requirement

The normal loss of fluid through the skin, respiratory tract, faeces and urine accounts for 2.5–3 litres per day in an average adult, or approximately 1.5 ml/kg/hour. It is proportionately greater in children.

The maintenance fluid requirement is increased:

- In hot climates
- The patient is pyrexial
- The patient has diarrhoea
- During preoperative fasting: 'nil by mouth'.

## NORMAL MAINTENANCE FLUIDS AND ELECTROLYTE REQUIREMENTS

| Weight | Fluid ml/kg/24 hours | Sodium mmol/kg/24 hours | Potassium mmol/kg/24 hours |
|---|---|---|---|
| **Children** | | | |
| First 10 kg | 100 (4*) | 3 | 2 |
| Second 10 kg | 50 (2*) | 1.5 | 1 |
| Subsequent kg | 20 (1*) | 0.75 | 0.5 |
| **Adults** | | | |
| All weights (kg) | 35 (1.5*) | 1 | 0.75 |

\* Fluid requirements in ml/kg/hour

## ADULT REPLACEMENT VOLUME REQUIREMENTS FOR PATIENTS UNDERGOING SURGERY

| Type of loss | Volume | Type of fluid |
|---|---|---|
| **Blood** | | |
| Up to allowable volume | 3 x volume lost | Crystalloid replacement fluid |
| **or** | 1 x volume lost | Colloid |
| When allowable volume exceeded | 1 x volume lost | Blood |
| **+ Other fluids** | | |
| Maintenance fluids | 1.5 ml/kg/hour | Crystalloid maintenance fluid |
| Maintenance deficit | 1.5 ml/kg/hour | Crystalloid maintenance fluid |
| Body cavity losses | 5 ml/kg/hour | Crystalloid maintenance fluid |
| Continuing losses | Measure | Crystalloid/colloid |

Adult replacement volume = Blood loss + other losses

## Preoperative fasting

Add the maintenance fluid deficit that occurs during preoperative fasting to the volume of replacement fluid.

## Body cavity losses

During a laparotomy or thoracotomy, replace the evaporation of water with 5 ml/kg/hour of fluid for each cavity opened, in addition to the maintenance fluid.

## Continuing losses

Measure any continuing fluid losses, such as nasogastric aspirate or drainage fluid, and add to the volume of replacement fluid.

# Blood transfusion strategies
## Blood ordering schedules

Blood ordering schedules aid clinicians to decide on the quantity of blood to crossmatch (or group and screen) for a patient about to undergo surgery (see example on pp. 172–173).

Blood ordering schedules should always be developed locally and should be used simply as a guide to expected normal blood usage (see p. 41).

Each hospital transfusion committee should agree a procedure for the prescribing clinician to override the blood ordering schedule when it is probable that the patient will need more blood than is stipulated: for example, if the procedure is likely to be more complex than usual or if the patient has a coagulation defect. In such cases, additional units of blood should be crossmatched as requested by the clinician.

## Group O RhD-negative blood

The availability in a hospital of two units of group O RhD-negative blood, reserved for use only in an emergency, can be a life-saving strategy.

Unused units should be regularly replaced well before their expiry date so they can enter the blood bank stock.

## Control of bleeding

When the decision is made to improve the oxygen-carrying capacity of the patient by means of a blood transfusion, maximize the benefits of the transfusion by transfusing blood when surgical bleeding is controlled, if possible.

## Massive or large volume transfusion

Patients who need large volumes of blood and intravenous fluids may have special problems. See pp. 74–77.

## EXAMPLE OF A BLOOD ORDERING SCHEDULE: A GUIDE TO EXPECTED NORMAL BLOOD USAGE FOR SURGICAL PROCEDURES IN ADULT PATIENTS

| Procedure | Action |
| --- | --- |
| **General surgery** | |
| Cholecystectomy | G & S |
| Laparotomy: planned exploration | G & S |
| Liver biopsy | G & S |
| Hiatus hernia | X-M 2 |
| Partial gastrectomy | G & S |
| Colectomy | X-M 2 |
| Mastectomy: simple | G & S |
| Mastectomy: radical | X-M 2 |
| Thyroidectomy: partial/total | X-M 2 (+ 2) |
| **Cardiothoracic** | |
| Angioplasty | G & S |
| Open heart surgery | X-M 4 (+ 4) |
| Bronchoscopy | G & S |
| Open pleural/lung biopsy | G & S |
| Lobectomy/pneumonectomy | X-M 2 |
| **Vascular** | |
| Aortic-iliac endarterectomy | X-M 4 |
| Femoral endarterectomy | G & S |
| Femoro-popliteal bypass | G & S |
| Ilio-femoral bypass | X-M 2 |
| Resection abdminal aortic aneurysm | X-M 6 (+ 2) |
| **Neurosurgery** | |
| Craniotomy, craniectomy | |
| Meningioma | G & S |
| Head injury, extradural haematoma | X-M 4 |
| Vascular surgery (aneurysms, | G & S |
|    A-V malformations) | X-M 3 |
| **Urology** | |
| Ureterolithotomy | G & S |
| Cystotomy | G & S |
| Ureterolithotomy & cystotomy | G & S |
| Cystectomy | X-M 4 |

| Procedure | Action |
|---|---|
| Open nephrolithotomy | X-M 2 |
| Open prostatectomy (RPP) | X-M 2 |
| Transurethral resection prostatectomy (TURP) | G & S |
| Renal transplantation | X-M 2 |

**Obstetrics & gynaecology**

| | |
|---|---|
| Termination of pregnancy | G & S |
| Normal delivery | G & S |
| Caesarean section | G & S |
| Placenta praevia/retained placenta | X-M 4 |
| Antepartum/postpartum haemorrhage | X-M 2 |
| Dilatation & curettage | G & S |
| Hysterectomy: abdominal or vaginal: simple | G & S |
| Hysterectomy: abdominal or vaginal: extended | X-M 2 |
| Myomectomy | X-M 2 |
| Hydatidiform mole | X-M 2 |
| Oophorectomy (radical) | X-M 4 |

**Orthopaedics**

| | |
|---|---|
| Disc surgery | G & S |
| Laminectomy | G & S |
| Removal hip pin or femoral nail | G & S |
| Total hip replacement | X-M 2 (+ 2) |
| Ostectomy/bone biopsy (except upper femur) | G & S |
| Nailing fractured neck of femur | G & S |
| Laminectomy | G & S |
| Internal fixation of femur | X-M 2 |
| Internal fixation: tibia or ankle | G & S |
| Arthroplasty: total hip | X-M 3 |
| Spinal fusion (scoliosis) | X-M 2 |
| Spinal decompression | X-M 2 |
| Peripheral nerve surgery | G & S |

X-M = Crossmatch       G & S = ABO/Rh group and antibody screen

(+ ) indicates additional units may be required, depending on surgical complications

## Autologous blood transfusion

Autologous transfusion involves the collection and subsequent reinfusion of the patient's own blood or blood products.

It should only be considered where sufficient blood loss to require a transfusion has occurred or is anticipated to occur although, in emergency, it may be the only readily available source of blood for transfusion. Get advice from the blood bank.

Different methods of autologous transfusion can be used alone or in combination to reduce or eliminate the need for allogeneic blood.

### Preoperative blood donation

Preoperative blood donation involves the collection and storage of the patient's own blood prior to elective surgery.

1  A unit of the patient's own blood is collected every five or more days in the period leading up to surgery.

2  The blood is tested, labelled and stored to the same standard as allogeneic blood and the patient is prescribed oral iron supplements.

3  On the date of operation, up to 4–5 units of stored blood are then available if transfusion becomes necessary during the procedure.

#### Disadvantages

■  Requires considerable planning and organization

■  Initial costs can be higher than allogeneic transfusion

■  Criteria for patient eligibility must be defined: some patients are not fit enough or live too far away from the hospital to make repeated donations

■  Does not avoid the risk of bacterial contamination as a result of collection or storage problems

■  Does not reduce the risk of procedural errors that can cause incompatibility of blood.

Unused units of the blood should not be transferred to the allogeneic pool for the benefit of other patients unless they have been tested for various disease markers, such as HBsAg and anti-HIV.

# Acute normovolaemic haemodilution

Acute preoperative normovolaemic haemodilution involves:

- The removal of a predetermined volume of the patient's own blood immediately prior to the commencement of surgery
- Its simultaneous replacement with sufficient crystalloid or colloid fluids to maintain the blood volume.

During surgery, the haemodiluted patient will lose fewer red cells for a given blood loss and the autologous blood collected can subsequently be reinfused, preferably when surgical bleeding has been controlled.

The fresh units of autologous blood will contain a full complement of coagulation factors and platelets.

## Precautions

1. Exclude unsuitable patients, such as those who cannot compensate for the reduction in oxygen supply due to haemodilution.

2. Carefully assess the volume of blood to be removed and replace with crystalloid (at least 3 ml for every 1 ml blood collected), or colloid (1 ml for every 1 ml collected).

3. Monitor the patient carefully and maintain blood volume and oxygen delivery at all times, particularly when surgical blood loss occurs.

# Blood salvage

Blood salvage is the collection of shed blood from a wound, body cavity or joint space and its subsequent reinfusion into the same patient. It can be used both during elective surgery (e.g. cardiothoracic procedures) and in emergency or trauma surgery (e.g. ruptured ectopic pregnancy or ruptured spleen).

## Contraindications

1. Blood contaminated with bowel contents, bacteria, fat, amniotic fluid, urine, malignant cells or irrigants: however, where salvage is being performed as an emergency, these risks must be balanced against the life-saving benefits to the patient.

2. Reinfusion of salvaged blood which has been shed for more than 6 hours: the transfusion is likely to be harmful since there will be haemolysis of red cells, hyperkalaemia and a risk of bacterial contamination.

## Methods of blood salvage

### Gauze filtration

This method is inexpensive and suitable for the salvage of blood from body cavities.

1   At operation and using an aseptic technique, collect blood from the cavity using a ladle or small bowl.

2   Mix the blood with anticoagulant.

3   Filter the blood through gauze and reinfuse into the patient.

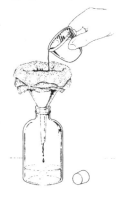

### Manual suction collection system

Commercially available suction systems incorporate suction tubing connected to a specially designed storage bottle containing anticoagulant.

1   At operation, blood is sucked from the cavity or wound directly into the bottle.

2   In certain circumstances, blood may also be collected postoperatively via surgical drains using this method.

3   Suction pressure should be as low as possible to avoid haemolysis of red cells.

### Automated suction collection systems

These commercially available systems, often called cell-savers, collect, anticoagulate, wash, filter, and re-suspend red cells in crystalloid fluid prior to reinfusion.

Although a significant amount of automation is involved in the process, a dedicated operator of the device is frequently required. The high capital cost of this equipment, together with the significant cost of disposable items for each patient, may limit its availability.

# Care in the postoperative period

**Monitoring**

- Monitor particularly for clinical signs of hypovolaemia and blood loss
- Regularly check wound and drains for haematoma and bleeding
- Check abdominal girth measurements.

**Postoperative oxygen**

- Give supplementary oxygen to all patients recovering from a general anaesthetic.

**Fluid balance to maintain normovolaemia**

- Give intravenous fluids to replace losses and maintenance requirements
- Continue until oral intake is adequate and postoperative bleeding is unlikely.

**Analgesia**

Postoperative pain is a major cause of hypertension and restlessness and can aggravate bleeding and increase blood loss:

- Give adequate analgesia throughout the perioperative period
- Where surgery involves a limb, elevate it postoperatively to reduce swelling, control venous blood loss and reduce pain.

**Surgical re-exploration**

Consider early surgical re-exploration where significant blood loss continues to occur postoperatively and there is no treatable disturbance of the coagulation status of the patient.

**Postoperative transfusions**

The use of intravenous fluids can cause haemodilution and lower the haemoglobin concentration. This alone is not an indication for transfusion.

Transfuse only if the patients has clinical signs and symptoms of hypoxia and/or a continued substantial blood loss.

**Haematinics**

Give iron supplements (ferrous sulphate: 200 mg tid) in the later postoperative period to help restore the haemoglobin level.

# Notes

# Acute surgery & trauma

## Key points

The immediate management of all seriously-ill patients should be carried out in the following three phases.

**Phase 1: ASSESS AND RESUSCITATE**
Follow the ABC sequence.

A Airway control
- Assess patient
- Establish a patent airway
- Stabilize cervical spine

B Breathing
- Assess patient
- Administer high concentrations of oxygen
- Assist ventilation, if indicated
- Alleviate tension pneumothorax or massive haemothorax
- Seal open pneumothorax

C Circulation and control of haemorrhage
- Direct pressure to bleeding site
- Assess patient
- Intravenous access and blood samples
- Fluid resuscitation
- Transfusion, if indicated

D Disorders of the central nervous system
- Determine level of consciousness
- Assess localizing neurological signs

E Exposure
- Completely undress the patient
- Urinary and nasogastric catheters

## Phase 2: REASSESS

Evaluate the response to resuscitation

- Assess pulse, blood pressure, capillary refill time
- Assess urine output
- Assess central venous pressure changes
- Assess acid-base balance

Plan a management strategy based on the rate of response to initial fluid administration

- Rapid response
- Transient response
- No response

Perform a detailed examination

- Head-to-toe examination if patient is stabilized (secondary survey)

## Phase 3: DEFINITIVE TREATMENT

Implement the management strategy and prepare the patient for definitive treatment

- Surgery
- Conservative treatment

The basic principles of resuscitation and management apply to paediatric patients.

# Assessment and resuscitation

## A Airway control

1 Ensure the patient has a clear, unobstructed airway.

2 Noisy or laboured breathing or paradoxical respiratory movements indicate airway obstruction.

3 Remove vomit, blood or foreign material from the mouth.

4 Lift the chin of an unconscious patient to prevent obstruction of the airway by the tongue.

5 Other measures to secure airway, if necessary:
- Forward jaw thrust
- Insert oro/nasopharyngeal airway
- Endotracheal intubation
- Cricothyroid puncture
- Tracheostomy.

6 Immobilize neck with rigid collar if cervical spine injury is suspected, or hold patient's head in a neutral position.

7 Stabilize neck while clearing airway or inserting tube.

## B Breathing

1 Check for injuries to thorax.

2 Measure respiratory rate.

3 Give assisted ventilation if the patient is not breathing or has inadequate respiration.

4 Give high concentrations of oxygen.

5 Examine the respiratory system to exclude a tension pneumothorax or massive haemothorax.

6 If present, treat immediately by pleural drainage with an underwater seal.

7 Seal an open chest wound.

## C Circulation and control of haemorrhage

1 Control haemorrhage:
- Control extensive bleeding by pressure on bleeding site

- Tourniquets are not recommended as they may increase tissue destruction
- Leave penetrating objects in-situ until surgical exploration.

2 Assess cardiovascular system
- Pulse rate
- Capillary refill time (the time taken for colour to return to the finger pad or nailbed after it has been briefly compressed; greater than 2 seconds is abnormal)
- Level of consciousness
- Blood pressure.

3 Assess hypovolaemia
- Estimate blood or fluid losses from the patient's clinical signs and the nature of injury or surgical condition
- Concealed bleeding is difficult to assess. Do not underestimate blood loss:
  — Closed fractured femur: up to 2000 ml
  — Fractured pelvis: up to 3000 ml
  — Ruptured spleen or ectopic pregnancy: total blood volume can be lost very rapidly
- Soft tissue injury and tissue oedema contribute to hypovolaemia.

## D Disorders of the central nervous system

1 Check conscious level: blood loss >30% reduces cerebral perfusion and unconsciousness results.

2 Check pupil response to light.

3 Grade the patient as:
  A **A**lert
  V Responds to **V**erbal commands
  P Responds to **P**ainful stimuli
  U **U**nresponsive

## E Expose and examine the whole body

1 Remove all clothing of trauma casualties to allow a thorough survey of injuries.

2 Keep patient warm.

3 Insert urinary catheter.

4 Consider nasogastric tube, especially in children, unless a fracture of anterior cranial fossa is suspected.

# Hypovolaemia

Hypovolaemia can be classified into four classes, based on the patient's clinical signs and assuming the normal blood volume of an adult to be 70 ml/kg.

This is a useful guide, but patients may not fit a precise class and variations will occur.

A patient's response to hypovolaemia is influenced by:

- Age
- Medical disorders: e.g. diabetes, ischaemic heart disease, renal failure, pre-eclampsia
- Medications.

| CLASSIFICATION OF HYPOVOLAEMIA IN THE ADULT | | | | |
|---|---|---|---|---|
| | Class I Mild | Class II Progressing | Class III Severe | Class IV End stage |
| % of blood volume lost | <15% | 15–30% | 30–40% | >40% |
| Volume lost in 70 kg adult | <750 ml | 750–1500 ml | 1500–2000 ml | >2000 ml |
| Pulse rate | Normal | >100 | >120 | >140 but variable in terminal stages of shock |
| Pulse pressure | Normal | Reduced | Very reduced | Very reduced/ absent |
| Systolic blood pressure | Normal | Normal | Reduced | Very reduced |
| Capillary refill | Normal | Prolonged | Very prolonged | Absent |
| Respiratory rate | Normal | 20–30 | 30–40 | >45 or slow sighing respiration |
| Mental state | Alert | Anxious | Confused | Comatosed/ unconscious |
| Urine output | >30 ml/hr | 20–30 ml/hr | 5–20 ml/hr | < 5 ml/hr |

## Intravenous access

1 Insert two cannulae (14 g or 16 g in an adult or the appropriate size in a child) in the antecubital fossae or any large peripheral vein (see pp. 185–186). Always wear gloves when performing intravenous cannulation.

2 Do not put IV lines in injured limbs.

3 If intravenous access is not possible, cannulate the external jugular vein or femoral vein.

4 Alternatively, consider a venous cutdown (see p. 187–188).

5 Central venous access (see p. 189–190) is rarely indicated for initial resuscitation, but may later be useful as a guide to fluid replacement. Catheterization of the internal jugular vein should only be performed by a trained person.

6 Take blood samples for haematology, biochemistry and compatibility testing.

## Fluid resuscitation

1 Give intravenous fluids within minutes of admission to hospital to restore the circulating blood volume rapidly and maintain organ perfusion.

2 Infuse normal saline (sodium chloride 0.9%) or a balanced salt solution as rapidly as possible in a volume at least three times the volume lost in order to correct hypovolaemia.

3 Alternatively, give colloid solutions in volumes equal to the blood loss as they remain within the circulation for longer.

4 Do not use dextrose or other solutions with a low sodium content unless there is no alternative.

5 Give initial fluid bolus of 20–30 ml/kg of crystalloid, or 10–20 ml/kg of colloid, over 5 minutes to any patient showing signs of more than 15% blood loss (Class II hypovolaemia and above). Where possible, the fluid should be warmed to prevent further patient cooling.

6 Assess the patient's response to guide further fluid infusion.

7 If urgent transfusion is likely to be life-saving, do not wait for fully crossmatched blood, but use uncrossmatched group O negative blood or uncrossmatched blood of the same ABO and RhD group as the patient.

## Intravenous cannulation

Cephalic vein    Basilic vein    Forearm vein    Great saphenous vein    Scalp veins

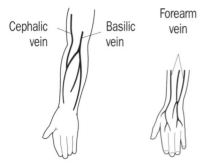
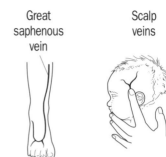

1 Occlude the venous drainage with a tourniquet or finger pressure. This will allow the vein to fill and stand out. Tap the vein to make it stand out.

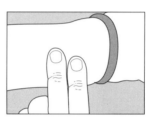

2 Identify a vein, preferably with a Y-junction. Stretch the skin below the vein. This will stop it moving.

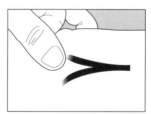

3 Gently push the needle through the skin at the Y-junction. Do not go too deep. Always wear gloves when performing intravenous cannulation.

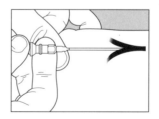

4 Stop pushing when blood appears in the cannula.

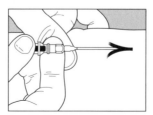

## Intravenous cannulation

5 Hold the needle steady and push the cannula up the vein.

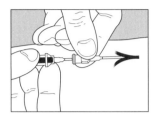

6 When the cannula is fully in the vein, release the tourniquet and remove the needle.

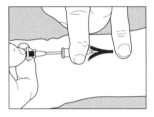

7 Connect up to the drip set.

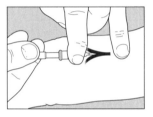

8 Fix the cannula with strapping.

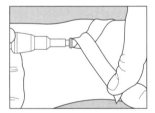

## Sites for venous cutdown

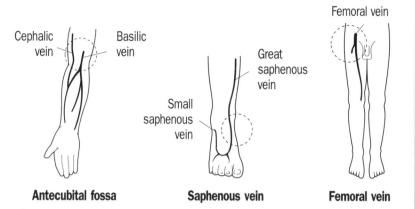

**Antecubital fossa**

Cephalic vein · Basilic vein

**Saphenous vein**

Great saphenous vein · Small saphenous vein

**Femoral vein**

Femoral vein

1 Infiltrate the skin with local anaesthetic.

2 Make a transverse incision.

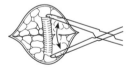

3 Expose the vein.

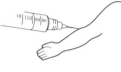

4 Insert sutures loosely at the proximal and distal ends of the vein.

## Sites for venous cutdown

5 Make a small
 incision in the vein.

6 Expose the opening in
 the vein and insert the
 cannula.

7 Tie the upper suture
 to secure cannula.

8 Close the wound.

# Sites for central venous catheterization

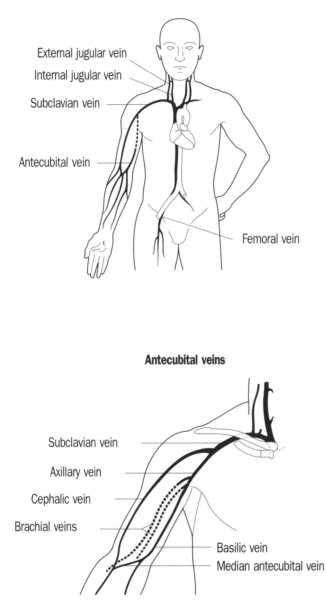

External jugular vein

Internal jugular vein

Subclavian vein

Antecubital vein

Femoral vein

## Antecubital veins

Subclavian vein

Axillary vein

Cephalic vein

Brachial veins

Basilic vein

Median antecubital vein

The basilic vein takes a smoother
course than the cephalic and is
often the most successful approach

## Sites for central venous catheterization

**Femoral vein**

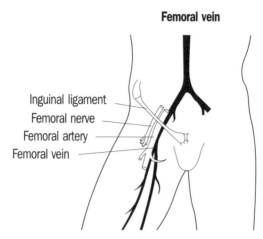

Inguinal ligament
Femoral nerve
Femoral artery
Femoral vein

The skin is entered at a 45° angle 3 cm below the inguinal ligament and 1 cm medial to the maximal femoral artery pulsation.

**Internal jugular vein**
Identify the point midway between a line joining the mastoid and sternal notch. Insert the needle at a 45° angle just lateral to this point and aim the needle at the nipple.

**External jugular vein**
In the head-down position, the external jugular vein will fill and become visible. It can then be cannulated in the normal way. This vein is extremely useful for fluid resuscitation and can often be found when others have collapsed.

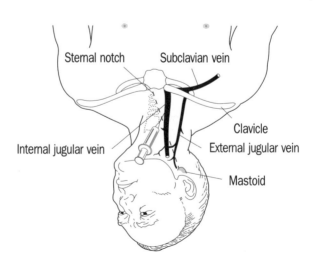

Sternal notch
Internal jugular vein

Subclavian vein
Clavicle
External jugular vein
Mastoid

## Reassessment

### Evaluate the response to resuscitation

1 Reassess the patient's clinical condition.

2 Detect any change in the patient's condition.

3 Assess patient's response to resuscitation.

#### Signs of normovolaemia being re-established

- Decreasing heart rate
- Reduced capillary refill time
- Return of peripheral pulses
- Increasing urine output
- Normalizing arterial pH
- Return of normal blood pressure
- Improving conscious level
- Slow rise in CVP

### Management strategy

The management strategy should be based on the patient's response to initial resuscitation and fluid administration.

#### 1 Rapid improvement

Some patients respond quickly to the initial fluid bolus and remain stable after it is completed. These patients have usually lost less than 20% of their blood volume.

#### 2 Transient improvement

Patients who have lost 20–40% of their blood volume or are still bleeding will improve with the initial fluid bolus, but circulation deteriorates when fluid is slowed.

#### 3 No improvement

Failure to respond to adequate volumes of fluids and blood requires immediate surgical intervention to control exsanguinating haemorrhage.

In trauma, a failure to respond may also be due to heart failure caused by myocardial contusion or cardiac tamponade.

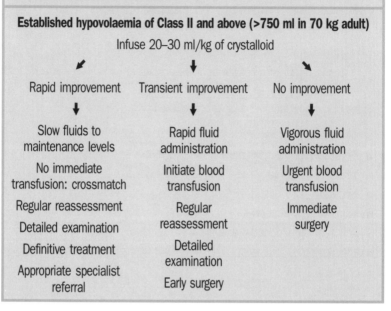

**MANAGEMENT STRATEGY IN THE ADULT BASED ON RATE OF RESPONSE TO INITIAL FLUID ADMINISTRATION**

Established hypovolaemia of Class II and above (>750 ml in 70 kg adult)

Infuse 20–30 ml/kg of crystalloid

| Rapid improvement | Transient improvement | No improvement |
|---|---|---|
| Slow fluids to maintenance levels | Rapid fluid administration | Vigorous fluid administration |
| No immediate transfusion: crossmatch | Initiate blood transfusion | Urgent blood transfusion |
| Regular reassessment | Regular reassessment | Immediate surgery |
| Detailed examination | Detailed examination | |
| Definitive treatment | Early surgery | |
| Appropriate specialist referral | | |

Patients who show no improvement following initial fluid administration or in whom there is obvious exsanguinating haemorrhage require urgent surgery, together with resuscitation.

## Detailed examination

Perform a detailed examination as soon as the patient is stabilized.

1 Obtain any history that may be available from the patient or relatives.

2 Carry out detailed head-to-toe examination.

3 Arrange X-rays or other investigations required.

4 Give tetanus immunization.

5 Decide on need for antibiotics.

6 Make a diagnosis.

It may only be possible to conduct the secondary survey after surgical control of exsanguinating haemorrhage.

# Definitive management

Definitive management of haemorrhage usually requires surgery. The aim is to achieve this within one hour of presentation, using techniques to conserve and manage blood loss during surgery (see pp. 162–164).

Administering large volumes of blood and intravenous fluids may give rise to complications (see pp. 74–77).

# Other causes of hypovolaemia

Hypovolaemia due to medical and surgical causes other than haemorrhage should be initially managed in a very similar way, with specific treatment (e.g. insulin, antibiotics) for the causative condition.

The need for blood transfusion and surgical intervention will depend on the diagnosis.

### Other causes of hypovolaemia

**Medical**
- Cholera
- Diabetic ketoacidosis
- Septic shock
- Acute adrenal insufficiency

**Surgical**
- Major trauma
- Severe burns
- Peritonitis
- Crush injury

# Paediatric patients

The principles of management and resuscitation are the same as for adults.

### Normal values for paediatric vital signs and blood volume

| Age | Pulse rate beats/minute | Blood pressure systolic mmHG | Respiratory rate breaths/minute | Blood volume ml/kg |
|---|---|---|---|---|
| <1 year | 120–160 | 70–90 | 30–40 | 85–90 |
| 1–5 years | 100–120 | 80–90 | 25–30 | 80 |
| 6–12 years | 80–100 | 90–110 | 20–25 | 80 |
| >12 years | 60–100 | 100–120 | 15–20 | 70 |

The normal blood volume is proportionately greater in children and is calculated at 80 ml/kg in a child and 85–90 ml/kg in the neonate.

Using a height/weight chart is often the easiest method of finding the approximate weight of a seriously-ill child.

## Venous access

1   Venous access is difficult in children, especially if they are hypovolaemic.

2   Useful sites for cannulation are:

- Long saphenous vein over ankle
- External jugular vein
- Femoral veins.

## Intraosseous infusion

1   The intraosseous route can provide the quickest access to the circulation in a shocked child if venous cannulation is impossible.

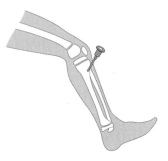

2   Fluids, blood and many drugs can be administered by this route.

3   Site the intraosseous needle in the anterior tibial plateau, 2–3 cm below the tibial tuberosity. Avoid the epiphysial growth plate.

4   Fluids may need to be administered under pressure or via a syringe when rapid replacement is required.

5   If special intraosseous needles are unavailable, use a spinal, epidural or bone marrow biopsy needle.

6   The intraosseous route can be used in all age groups, but is generally most successful in children below six years of age.

## Hypovolaemia

1  Recognizing hypovolaemia can be more difficult than in the adult.

2  Vital signs may change little, even when up to 25% of blood volume is lost (Class I and II hypovolaemia).

3  Tachycardia is often the earliest response to hypovolaemia, but can also be caused by fear or pain.

### CLASSIFICATION OF HYPOVOLAEMIA IN CHILDREN

|                       | Class I     | Class II    | Class III     | Class IV                  |
|-----------------------|-------------|-------------|---------------|---------------------------|
| Blood volume lost     | <15%        | 15–25%      | 25–40%        | >40%                      |
| Pulse rate            | Increased   | >150        | >150          | Increased or bradycardia  |
| Pulse pressure        | Normal      | Reduced     | Very reduced  | Absent                    |
| Systolic blood pressure | Normal    | Reduced     | Very reduced  | Unrecordable              |
| Capillary refill time | Normal      | Prolonged   | Very prolonged| Absent                    |
| Respiratory rate      | Normal      | Increased   | Increased     | Slow sighing respiration  |
| Mental state          | Normal      | Irritable   | Lethargic     | Comatosed                 |
| Urine output          | <1 ml/kg/hr | <1 ml/kg/hr | <1 ml/kg/hr   | <1 ml/kg/hr               |

## Replacement fluids

1  Initial fluid challenge in a child should represent 25% of blood volume as the signs of hypovolaemia may only become apparent after this amount is lost.

2  Give 20 ml/kg of crystalloid fluid to a child showing signs of Class II hypovolaemia or greater.

3  Depending on response, repeat up to three times (up to 60 ml/kg), if necessary.

## Transfusion

1  Children who have a transient response or no response to initial fluid challenge require further crystalloid fluids and blood transfusion.

2 Initially transfuse 20 ml/kg of whole blood or 10 ml/kg of packed cells.

## Hypothermia

1 Heat loss occurs rapidly in a child due to the high surface-to-mass ratio.

2 A child who is hypothermic may become refractory to treatment.

3 Maintain the body temperature.

## Gastric dilatation

1 Acute gastric dilatation is commonly seen in the seriously ill or injured child.

2 Gastric decompression, via a nasogastric tube.

## Analgesia

1 Give analgesic after initial fluid resuscitation, except in the case of head injury.

2 Give 50 $\mu$g/kg intravenous bolus of morphine, followed by 10–20 $\mu$g/kg increments at 10 minute intervals until an adequate response is achieved.

Tachycardia is earliest response to hypovolaemia

Gastric decompression via a nasogastric tube

Heat loss occurs rapidly; keep warm

Consider intraosseous route

Blood volume is 80 ml/kg in the child and 85–90 ml/kg in the neonate

Initially give 20 ml/kg of crystalloid replacement fluid if signs of hypovolaemia

# Notes

# Burns

## Key points

1 The early management of seriously burned patients is similar to the management of other trauma patients.

2 In common with other forms of hypovolaemia, the primary goal of treatment is to restore the circulating blood volume in order to maintain tissue perfusion and oxygenation.

3 Give intravenous fluids if the burn surface area is greater than 15% in an adult or greater than 10% in a child.

4 The use of crystalloid fluids alone is safe and effective for burns resuscitation. Using the correct amount of fluid in serious burns injuries is much more important than the type of fluid used.

5 The most useful indicator of fluid resuscitation is hourly monitoring of urine output. In the absence of glycosuria and diuretics, aim to maintain a urine output of 0.5 ml/kg/hour in adults and 1 ml/kg/hour in children.

6 Consider transfusion only if there are signs indicating inadequate oxygen delivery.

# Immediate management

The immediate management of seriously burned patients is similar to the management of other trauma patients (Airway, Breathing, Circulation, etc.).

## Special points

1 First aiders must first protect themselves from the source of danger: heat, smoke, chemical or electrical hazard.

2 Stop the burning process:
   - Evacuate patient from source of danger
   - Remove clothing
   - Wash chemical burns with large amounts of water.

3 Assess for airway injury:
   - Injury to upper airway injury can cause airway obstruction, but may not develop immediately
   - Give high concentrations of oxygen, endotracheal intubation and mechanical ventilation, if required
   - Frequent assessment of airway and ventilation is essential

   Endotracheal intubation may cause damage, especially when hot air has been inhaled. Consider the use of a laryngeal mask to avoid trauma.

4 Unconscious patients with electrical or lightning burns may be in ventricular fibrillation.

   External cardiac massage or defibrillation can be life-saving.

---

### Features of an airway injury

**Definite features**
- Pharyngeal burns
- Sooty sputum
- Stridor
- Hoarseness
- Airway obstruction
- Raised carboxyhaemoglobin level

**Suspicious features**
- History of confinement in burning area
- Singed eyebrows and nasal hair
- Cough
- Wheeze
- Respiratory crepitations

---

5   Cool the burned area with *large* amounts of cold water as soon as possible following the burn.

6   Seal phosphorus burns with soft paraffin (vaseline) or immerse in water to prevent reignition.

7   Remember:
   ■   There may be other injuries
   ■   Medical conditions, such as a cerebrovascular accident, may have caused a fall into a fire.

8   Intravenous fluids are required for burns:
   ■   >15% in an adult under 50 years of age
   ■   >10% in a child or adult over 50 years of age.

## Assessing the severity of the burn

Morbidity and mortality rise with increasing burned surface area. They also rise with increasing age so that even small burns may be fatal in elderly people.

Burns are considered serious if:
   ■   >15% in an adult
   ■   >10% in a child
   ■   The burned patient is very young or elderly.

### Estimating the burned surface area
#### Adults
The 'Rule of 9's' is commonly used to estimate the burned surface area in adults.

   ■   The body is divided into anatomical regions that represent 9% (or multiples of 9%) of the total body surface

   ■   The outstretched palm and fingers approximates to 1% of the body surface area. If the burned area is small, assess how many times your hand covers the area.

#### Children
The 'Rule of 9's' is too imprecise for estimating the burned surface area in children because the infant or young child's head and lower extremities represent different proportions of surface area than in an adult. Use the chart shown opposite to calculate the burned surface area in a child.

## Estimating the burned surface area in the adult

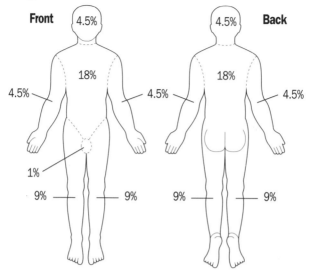

## Estimating the burned surface area in the child

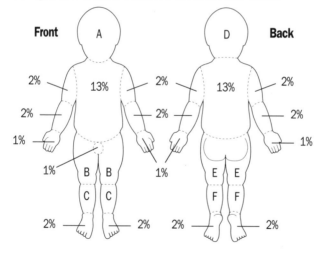

| Area | By age in years | | | |
|---|---|---|---|---|
| | **0** | **1** | **5** | **10** |
| Head (A/D) | 10% | 9% | 7% | 6% |
| Thigh (B/E) | 3% | 3% | 4% | 5% |
| Leg (C/F) | 2% | 3% | 3% | 3% |

# Estimating the depth of burn

Burns can be divided into three types. It is common to find all three types within the same burn wound and the depth may change with time, especially if infection supervenes. Any full thickness burn is serious.

| Depth of burn | Characteristics | Cause |
|---|---|---|
| First degree (superficial) burn | ■ Erythema<br>■ Pain<br>■ Absence of blisters | ■ Sunburn |
| Second degree or partial thickness burn | ■ Red or mottled<br>■ Swelling and blisters<br>■ Painful | ■ Contact with hot liquids<br>■ Flash burns |
| Third degree or full thickness burn | ■ Dark and leathery<br>■ Dry<br>■ Sensation only at edges | ■ Fire<br>■ Prolonged exposure to hot liquids/objects<br>■ Electricity or lightning |

## Other factors in assessing the severity of the burn

### Location/site of burn

Burns to the face, neck, hands, feet, perineum and circumferential burns (those encircling a limb, neck, etc.) are classified as serious.

### Other injuries

Inhalation injury, trauma or significant pre-existing illness increase risk.

### Criteria for hospitalization

- ■ >15% burns in an adult
- ■ >10% burns in a child
- ■ Any burn in the very young, the elderly or the infirm
- ■ Any full thickness burn
- ■ Burns of special regions: face, neck, hands, feet, perineum
- ■ Circumferential burns
- ■ Inhalation injury
- ■ Associated trauma or other pre-existing illness

# Fluid resuscitation

- Burning damages the capillaries
- Fluid leaks into the interstitial space, causing oedema
- Increased capillary permeability is not limited to the area of the burn, but affects the whole body
- Without treatment, hypovolaemia will cause reduced cardiac output, hypotension, oliguria and shock
- Capillary leakage arising from the burn site is greatest in the first 8 hours following injury and recovers after 18–36 hours.

**Treatment must restore the circulating blood volume in order to maintain tissue perfusion and oxygenation.**

## Calculating fluid requirements

1 Assess the severity of the burn
   - Ascertain the time of the burn injury
   - Estimate the weight of the patient
   - Estimate the % burned surface area.

2 Unless other injuries or conditions necessitate intravenous fluid replacement, commence oral fluids only if the % burned surface area is:
   - <15% in an adult
   - <10% in a child.

3 Give intravenous fluids if the burned surface area is:
   - >15% in an adult
   - >10% in a child.

4 Do not overestimate the burn size as this can result in fluid overload.

5 Calculate the fluid requirements from the time of burn injury.

6 During the first 48 hours, the use of a CVP line does not confer a particular advantage over more basic monitoring processes. This can later be reviewed if parenteral nutrition is involved.

## FORMULAE FOR CALCULATING FLUID REQUIREMENTS OF BURNS PATIENTS

### Adults

**First 24 hours**

Fluid required due to burn (ml) = 3 x weight (kg) x % burned area

*plus*

Fluid required for maintenance (ml) = 35 x weight (kg)

Give half this volume in the first 8 hours and the other half over the remaining 16 hours

**Second 24 hours**

Fluid required due to burn (ml) = 1 x weight (kg) x % burned area

*plus*

Fluid required for maintenance (ml) = 35 x weight (kg)

Give this volume over 24 hours

### Note

The upper limit of burned surface area is sometimes set at 45% for adults as a caution to avoid fluid overload. This limit can be overridden if indicated by the overall monitoring process.

### Children
**First 24 hours**

Fluid required due to burn (ml) = 3 x weight (kg) x % burned area

*plus*

Fluid required for maintenance (ml):

First 10 kg = 100 x weight (kg)

Second 10 kg = 75 x weight (kg)

Subsequent kg = 50 x weight (kg)

Give half this volume in the first 8 hours and the other half over the remaining 16 hours

### Note

1 The upper limit of burned surface area is sometimes set at 35% for children as a caution to avoid fluid overload. This limit can be overridden if indicated by the overall monitoring process.

2  In children, a very approximate weight guide is:

Weight (kg) = (Age in years + 4) x 2

Alternatively use a height/weight chart.

3  Children compensate for shock very well, but may then collapse rapidly.

4  Do not overestimate the burn size as this can result in fluid overload.

**EXAMPLE OF FLUID REQUIREMENTS FROM THE TIME OF INJURY:**
**Adult patient weighing 60 kg with 20% burn**

**First 24 hours**

| | |
|---|---|
| Replacement fluid: 3 x 60 (kg) x 20 (%) | 3600 ml |

*plus*

| | |
|---|---|
| Maintenance fluid: 35 x 60 (kg) | 2100 ml |
| Total fluid requirement | 5700 ml |

Give half this volume in the first 8 hours and the other half over the remaining 16 hours

**Second 24 hours**

| | |
|---|---|
| Replacement fluid: 1 x 60 (kg) x 20 (%) | 1200 ml |

*plus*

| | |
|---|---|
| Maintenance fluid: 35 x 60 (kg) | 2100 ml |
| Total fluid requirement | 3300 ml |

Give this volume over 24 hours

## Resuscitation fluids used in burns

1  Replace losses due to the burn with a **replacement** fluid, such as normal saline or a balanced salt solution: e.g. Hartmann's solution or Ringer's lactate.

2  Maintain patient's fluid balance with a **maintenance** fluid such as 4.3% dextrose in sodium chloride 0.18%.

3  Crystalloid fluids alone are safe and effective for burns resuscitation.

4  Colloid fluids are not required. There is no clear evidence that they significantly improve outcomes or reduce oedema formation when used as alternatives to crystalloids.

5   Using the correct amount of fluid in serious burns injuries is much more important than the type of fluid used.

**There is no justification for the use of blood in the early management of burns, unless other injuries warrant its use for red cell replacement.**

## Monitoring

1   Formulae for calculating fluid requirements should be used only a guide.

2   Regularly monitor and reassess the patient's clinical condition.

3   If necessary, adjust the volume of fluid given to maintain normovolaemia.

4   The most useful indicator of fluid resuscitation is hourly monitoring of urine output.

5   In the absence of glycosuria and diuretics, aim to maintain a urine output of 0.5 ml/kg/hour in adults and 1 ml/kg/hour in children.

6   Blood pressure can be difficult to ascertain in a severely burned patient and may be unreliable.

### Monitoring burns patients

- Blood pressure
- Heart rate
- Fluid input/output (hydration)
- Temperature
- Conscious level and anxiety state
- Respiratory rate/depth

## Continuing care of burns patients

1   Give anti-tetanus toxoid: it is essential for burned patients.

2   Give analgesia:
    - Initial 50 $\mu$g/kg intravenous bolus of morphine
    - Follow with 10–20 $\mu$g/kg increments at 10-minute intervals until the pain is just controlled

- Do not give intramuscular analgesics for 36 hours after the patient has been resuscitated
- Elevate burned limbs and cover partial thickness burns with clean linen to deflect air currents and reduce pain.

3 Insert nasogastric tube:
- If the patient has nausea or vomiting
- If the patient has abdominal distension
- If the burns involve more than 20% of the body area
- Use for feeding after 48 hours if patient cannot take food by mouth
- Use to administer antacids to protect the gastric mucosa.

4 Insert urinary catheter early to measure urine output.

5 Maintain room temperature above 28°C to reduce heat loss.

6 Control infection:
- Serious burns depress the immune system
- Infections and sepsis are common
- Use strict aseptic techniques when changing dressings and during invasive procedures
- Give antibiotics only for contaminated burns.

7 Maintain nutrition:
- Severe burns increase the body's metabolic rate, protein catabolism
- Weight loss and poor wound healing result
- Morbidity and mortality can be reduced by a high-protein, high calorie diet
- Feeding orally or via a nasogastric tube is safest
- Daily nutritional requirement of a severely burned patient is about 3 g/kg of protein and 90 calories/kg.

8 Anaemia:
- Minimize anaemia and hypoproteinaemia with high-protein, high-calorie diet with vitamin supplements and haematinics
- Consider blood transfusion only when there are signs of inadequate oxygen delivery.

9 Surgery:
- Debridement and skin grafting is often required for serious burns and can result in considerable blood loss

- Limit the area to be debrided at each procedure and use techniques to reduce operative blood loss.
- Give haematinics between surgical procedures
- Escharotomy (longitudinal splitting of deep circumferential burns to relieve swelling and pressure and restore the distal circulation) may also be urgently required to relieve airway compression resulting from circumferential chest burns.

    The procedure is painless and, if necessary, can be performed on the ward under sterile conditions.

10  Transfer seriously burned patients to specialized burns unit, if available:

- Transfer only following stabilization, usually after 36 hours or more.

11  Physiotherapy is vital to prevent pneumonia, disability and contracture formation. It must be started at an early stage.

# Notes

# Glossary

| | |
|---|---|
| Activated partial thromboplastin time (APTT) | A test of the blood coagulation system. Prolonged by plasma deficiency of coagulation factors XII, XI, IX, VIII, X, V, II and fibrinogen. Also referred to as partial thromboplastin time (kaolin) (PTTK). |
| Additive solution (red cell additive solution) | Proprietary formulas designed for reconstitution of red cells after separation of the plasma to give optimal red cell storage conditions. All are saline solutions with additions: e.g. adenine, glucose and mannitol. |
| Albumin | The main protein in human plasma. |
| Anti-D immunoglobulin | Human immunoglobulin G preparation containing a high level of antibody to the RhD antigen. |
| Balanced salt solution | Usually a sodium chloride salt solution with an electrolyte composition that resembles that of extracellular fluid: e.g. Ringer's lactate, Hartmann's solution. |
| Colloid solution | A solution of large molecules which have a restricted passage through capillary membranes. Used as an intravenous replacement fluid. Colloid solutions include gelatins, dextrans and hydroxyethyl starch. |
| Crystalloid solution | Aqueous solution of small molecules which easily pass through capillary membranes: e.g. normal saline, balanced salt solutions. |
| Decompensated anaemia | Severe clinically significant anaemia: anaemia with a haemoglobin level so low that oxygen transport is inadequate, even with all the normal compensatory responses operating. |
| Desferrioxamine | An iron-chelating (binding) agent that increases excretion of iron. |
| Dextran | A macromolecule consisting of a glucose solution that is used in some synthetic colloid solutions. |
| Disseminated intravascular coagulation (DIC) | Activation of the coagulation and fibrinolytic systems, leading to deficiencies of coagulation factors, fibrinogen and platelets. Fibrin degradation products are found in the blood. |

May also cause tissue/oxygen damage due to obstruction of small vessels. Clinically, often characterized by microvascular bleeding.

| | |
|---|---|
| Fibrin degradation products | Fragments of fibrin molecule formed by the action of fibrinolytic enzymes. Elevated levels in the blood are a feature of disseminated intravascular coagulation. |
| Fibrinogen | The major coagulant protein in plasma. Converted to (insoluble) fibrin by the action of thrombin. |
| Gelatin | A polypeptide of bovine origin that is used in some synthetic colloid solutions. |
| Haematocrit (Hct) | An equivalent measure to packed cell volume, derived by automated haematology analyses from the red cell indices. *See* Packed cell volume. |
| HLA | Human leucocyte antigen. |
| Hypochromia | Reduced iron content in red cells, indicated by reduced staining of the red cell. A feature of iron deficiency anaemia. *See* microcytosis. |
| Hypovolaemia | Reduced circulating blood volume. |
| Immunoglobulin (Ig) | Protein produced by B-lymphocytes and plasma cells. All antibodies are immunoglobulins. The main classes of immunoglobulin are IgG, IgM (mainly in plasma), IgA (protects mucosal surfaces) and IgE (causes allergic reactions). |
| International normalized ratio (INR) | Measures the anticoagulant effect of warfarin. Sometimes called the prothrombin time (PT). |
| Kernicterus | Damage to the basal ganglia of the brain, caused by fat-soluble bilirubin. Causes spasticity. Can be caused by haemolytic disease of the newborn. |
| Kleihauer test | Acid elution of blood film to allow counting of fetal red cells in maternal blood. |
| Macrocytosis | Red cells larger than normal. A feature of the red cells in, for example, anaemia due to deficiency of folic acid, vitamin $B_{12}$. |
| Maintenance fluids | Crystalloid solutions that are used to replace normal physiological losses through skin, lung, faeces and urine. |
| Megaloblasts | Precursors of abnormal red cells. Usually due to deficiency of vitamin $B_{12}$ and/or folate and develop into macrocytic red cells (enlarged red cells). |

| | |
|---|---|
| Microcytosis | Red cells smaller than normal. A feature of iron deficiency anaemia. *See also* Hypochromia. |
| Normal saline | An isotonic 0.9% sodium chloride solution. |
| Normovolaemia | Normal circulating blood volume. |
| Packed cell volume | Determined by centrifuging a small sample of blood in an anticoagulated capillary tube and measuring the volume of packed red cells as a percentage of the total volume. *See also* Haematocrit. |
| Plasma derivative | Human plasma protein prepared under pharmaceutical manufacturing conditions. Includes albumin, immunoglobulin and coagulation factor VIII and IX products. |
| Prothrombin time (PT) | A test of the blood clotting system. Prolonged by deficiencies of coagulation factors VIII, X, V, II and fibrinogen. *See* International normalized ratio. |
| Partial thromboplastin time (kaolin) (PTTK) | *See* Activated partial thromboplastin time (APTT). |
| Red cell components | Any blood component containing red cells: e.g. red cell concentrate, red cells in additive solution, packed red cells. |
| Red cell indices | Mean cell volume (MCV); mean cell haemoglobin (MCH); mean cell haemoglobin concentration (MCHC). |
| Refractory | A poor response to platelet transfusion. The patient's platelet count fails to rise by at least $10 \times 10^9$/L 18–24 hours after a platelet transfusion. Usually due to a clinical factor: e.g. fever, infection, DIC, splenomegaly, antibiotics. Also occurs if the platelet components transfused are defective. |
| Replacement fluids | Fluids used to replace abnormal losses of blood, plasma or other extracellular fluids by increasing the volume of the vascular compartment. Used to treat hypovolaemia and to maintain a normal blood volume. |
| Reticulocytes | Young red cells that still contain some RNA. Indicate increased rate of red cell production by bone marrow. |
| RhD | The most immunogenic antigen of the Rh blood group system. Antibodies to RhD are an important cause of haemolytic disease of the newborn. |

# Index